HOW TO BE WRINKLE-FREE

HOW TO BE WRINKLE-FREE

Look Younger Longer Without Plastic Surgery

CARLOTTA KARLSON JACOBSON,
Beauty Editor of <u>Harper's Bazaar</u>

with Catherine Ettlinger

Photography by Priscilla Rattazzi

G. P. Putnam's Sons/New York

G. P. Putnam's Sons
Publishers Since 1838
200 Madison Avenue
New York, NY 10016

Library of Congress Cataloging-in-Publication Data

Jacobson, Carlotta Karlson.
How to be wrinkle-free.

1. Skin—Wrinkles. 2. Skin—Aging. 3. Skin—Care and hygiene.
4. Beauty, Personal.
I. Ettlinger, Catherine.
II. Title. [DNLM: 1. Aging—popular works.
2. Dermatology—popular works.   WR 100 J17h]
RL87.J33   1986   646.7'26   85-19413
ISBN 0-399-13097-7

Printed in the United States of America

1   2   3   4   5   6   7   8   9   10

To Benjamin and Nicky, and my parents
for their enthusiasm and support
—C.K.J.

To Ralph, Rena and Nancy
—C.E.

ACKNOWLEDGMENTS

We want to thank all the people who gave us their time and expertise—and were absolutely crucial to making this book happen.

A very special thank you to: all the doctors and skin-care experts we consulted; the hair and makeup artists who did the makeovers—Garren, Sandy Linter, Louis Licari, Gad Cohen, Craig Gadson, Pablo Manzoni, Aldo Giacomello, Cida Nery and Francois Ilnseher; Dorothy Handelman, who did many of the photographs; Margaret A. Hinders, who did the line drawings; Charles Nicholas, who conceived of and illustrated the hair sketches; Antonio Lopez, who did the makeup and hair illustrations; Joan Harting, our friend, who let us photograph her; Lisa Klein and Jennifer Paley, who contributed every step of the way, and the rest of our friends who were always there to lend a helping hand; Cynthia Pillow, who deciphered the original manuscript and typed the first draft in record time; Just Loomis, who kindly photographed us for the jacket; and, of course, to *Harper's Bazaar* and *Mademoiselle*, our respective magazines, which provided us with the invaluable experience that enabled us to finally write this book.

CONTENTS

HOW TO BE

WRINKLE-FREE

AND SO IT STARTS:

WHY A BOOK ON

WRINKLES?

A day rarely goes by when someone doesn't ask me about wrinkles: What kinds of creams should I be using? Are there any professional treatments that really work to stave off lines? How should I change my makeup: Should I be using less, more or different colors altogether? What should I do with my hair—it's graying and I think it's adding years on to my looks. How can I be outdoors—whether it's just walking on the beach, gardening, playing tennis or skiing—and avoid sun damage to my skin?

Women are obsessive about wrinkles. No matter how much better they may feel about getting older—thanks to the women's movement and the recent popularity of such stars as Joan Collins and Jane Fonda—they still don't want to look old.

From beauty surveys I know that every woman's number-one priority when it comes to her looks is preventing wrinkles. Every woman—from twenty to sixty and beyond—wants to be wrinkle-free regardless of the time, energy or money (or sacrifice!) it takes. Women feel that the more youthful they look, the more successful they'll be in both their personal and professional lives.

I think the incredible popularity of *Harper's Bazaar's* annual "Over 40" issue is testimony to all this. The women we photograph every year are featured not only because they look great at forty-plus but because they're equally proud of how they look and what they've accomplished. (I have to laugh when I remember how I felt when I first went to *Harper's Bazaar* ten years ago and produced a small section for the woman over forty for the first time ever. I was terrified to ask celebrities and socialites to be in the section—who'd want to admit to the world that she was over forty? And this was only a decade ago!)

How things have changed! Women want advice and information about the aging process. They're what I call healthily narcissistic: They want to make taking care of themselves a way of life. That way of life has been my life and livelihood for almost fifteen years, and in that time I've accumulated a wealth of information on how to look beautiful, from the top experts all over the world.

In all honesty, I'm always amazed that for every question about wrinkles and the aging process, I seem to have the answer, some new tidbit of information that's just come across my desk—what will work; what won't. I've realized that I'm a veritable gold mine of information about wrinkles and skin care! Even the top executives from cosmetics companies here and abroad come to me: What treatment products do women want? What are women's biggest skin problems? Which of these problems are the companies failing to address? And I have answers for them, too.

I thought, I'm sharing information with my readers, colleagues and friends; why not share it with others, too? Why not catalogue everything I've learned? Why not, indeed?

In summary, then, here's why I decided to go ahead.

- First, because almost without exception *every woman's number-one beauty concern is aging*. Most women want to know how to stay younger-looking longer, and I know what to tell them.
- Second, because with all the beauty books glutting stores across the country, *there is no book (until now!) that is devoted entirely to wrinkles—women's biggest beauty priority*.

• And third, because I *want to set the record straight on the misinformation many women have accumulated about the aging process and what they can—and can't—do to hold back the hands of time and* look younger longer. Some women, for example, think there's nothing they can do about wrinkles—either you've got them or you don't; others think if they go for the works—if they use every cream and lotion, never go out in the sun, have facials every month—they can prevent wrinkles alto-gether and look young forever. While neither notion is entirely right or wrong, I felt that such misconceptions should be struck from the record once and for all. In this book I will provide a much-needed, realistic wrinkle-fighting program adaptable to any—and all—women's needs.

I asked Catherine Ettlinger, formerly a writer at *Bazaar*, now the managing editor of *Mademoiselle*, to help me. Our relationship, which was founded on professional respect, has grown into a great friendship. We are as different as we are alike in so many ways, and it's this dynamic that makes us work together so well: We are great complements to one another; great inspira-tions, too.

And we have developed the same basic personal and professional philos-ophy about aging: Wrinkles are a major problem—they may not be life threatening in the purest sense, but the stress and anxiety they produce can alter (if not threaten) the quality of life. You will wrinkle—that's a fact of life—but how much and when is all within your control. It's easy to look your best for your age—that's our goal, not to look years younger. The point is, you do not have to accept your face as is. You can smooth existing lines, prevent others from turning up altogether—and you can do it without plastic surgery if you know what to expect, what to look for and how to deal with aging as it progresses.

ONE

WHAT MAKES OLD

SKIN LOOK OLDER

FINDING YOUR PERSONAL WRINKLE PROFILE

To fully understand how to be wrinkle-free, you should have a basic knowledge of the composition of skin. None of this information is going to help you directly prevent wrinkles, but the better educated you are, the better equipped you'll be to do so. Plus, understanding the skin itself will help you better understand a lot of what you'll be reading in the upcoming chapters as well as what you're reading in magazines and on treatment-product labels.

So, in case you don't already know them by name and/or description, here are the various components of the skin, layer by layer, beginning on the outside and working in.

The *epidermis* is what you see. The outermost layer, it's the one that's affected by treatment products and makeup, the one that you can visibly change.

As thin as a sheet of paper, the epidermis is made up of many layers of cells, each of which is constantly moving: The lowest layer (basal) is where new, fully hydrated cells form and mature before they move upward; once they reach the skin's surface they die and are shed, to be replaced by new healthy cells underneath. (That's why exfoliation, the sloughing off of dead surface skin cells, can turn dull, dry skin glowing and beautiful.)

The *stratum corneum* (or *stratum lucidum*) is technically the uppermost layer of the epidermis. Its importance in determining how your skin looks is key not only in providing the crucial moisture needed to keep the young cells below it healthy but also in providing a barrier protective for them.

The *dermis* contains the support system for the skin—the system of collagen and elastin fibers that give skin its elasticity and youthful appearance; nerve fibers; nutrient-carrying blood vessels; melanin, which gives skin its color; hair follicles; sweat glands; and oil (or sebaceous) glands, which produce sebum, a complex mixture of fats that, along with water moisture, keeps your skin moist and soft.

The *subcutaneous fat tissue* is immediately below your dermis. This tissue, which contains some supporting fibers and the larger blood vessels, naturally thins as you age. The result: sagging skin. Obviously the fatter you are, the more support tissue and the fewer wrinkles you'll have. But, unfortunately, as much as I'd like to make this a rationale for being overweight, I cannot.

Essentially, everyone has the same basic skin makeup. Why, then, logically speaking, do some people wrinkle more—and earlier—than others?

The operative word here is *basic*. True, everyone has the same basic skin makeup, but there are variables. One person's skin can be thicker than another's; it can be fattier; or it can contain more pigment-protecting melanin.

Just how much you're going to wrinkle—and when—has a lot to do with your individual skin makeup—that is, your heredity.

Consider your heredity:

If you're	You have	And your wrinkle profile is
Celtic, Nordic, Scandinavian	thin fair skin; pale eyes	high risk for early and excessive wrinkling, especially those with dry skin
Latin, Mediterranean, Middle Eastern	oily, medium-thin skin; dark eyes	medium risk for early and excessive wrinkling
Black	normal-dry, thick skin; dark eyes	most wrinkle resistant

To find out exactly how wrinkle-prone you are right now, take these two tests.

The mirror test. Place a hand mirror flat on a table. Look down.

1. What happens to your cheeks?
2. What happens to the curve between your chin and neck?
3. What does your jaw look like?

If (1) your cheeks sag and hang instead of staying taut and tight . . . if (2) your chin-to-neck curve softens instead of staying sharp . . . or if (3) your jaw broadens, becomes squarer instead of maintaining angular strength . . . then, indeed, you are showing the signs of aging.

Need some further corroboration? Take *the pinch test.* Simply pinch some skin from the top of your hand. Hold it for ten seconds. If it takes more than two to three seconds to ease back into place, it has definitely lost—and is probably rapidly continuing to lose—its youthful elasticity.

Awareness of your wrinkle potential can help you hold off wrinkling and, in some cases, prevent lines from becoming as bad as they might without proper care. Take, for example, fair-skinned blondes: Without special sun-care precautions, they can expect premature wrinkling; with them, they can hold off lines for up to ten extra years.

Of course, the bottom line is that you will wrinkle whether you're wrinkle-resistant or not. It's just a matter of when . . . when your skin will get older-looking. What makes skin look old? Other than heredity, there are three basic reasons: (1) it gets drier; (2) it gets saggier, more wrinkly; and (3) it loses its youthful glow.

WHY SKIN GETS DRIER

Dehydration

All skin types, even the oiliest, dry out with age.

When I refer to skin's moisture I'm talking about both its water and its oil content. Oil production (by the sebaceous glands) slows with age, creating a double whammy: Not only does skin lose a major source of lubrication, it loses its protective barrier—the layer of oil, or sebum, that forms on the

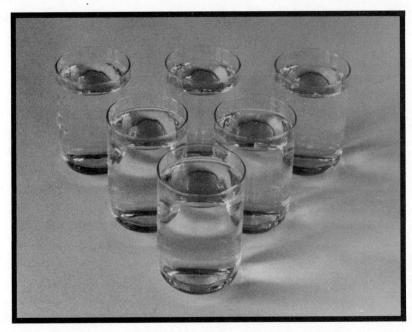

Dorothy Handelman

epidermis and locks in moisture. Thus, whatever water moisture your skin does have evaporates.

What this means: The older you get, the more conscious you're going to have to be about hydrating your skin. You'll have to drink more water—I recommend six to eight 8- to 10-ounce glasses a day if possible. Avoid diuretic foods, and, it should go without saying, avoid taking diuretic pills. Also, you'll have to step up your moisturizing routine.

Drop in Hormone Levels

Another element in the dehydration factor: As you age, your estrogen level drops, causing your skin to dry out. Later in Chapter 3, I'll go into the facts about topically applied hormones.

Overindulgence in Alcohol

Under normal circumstances your blood and skin tissue contain about 80 percent water, but when too much alcohol (a couple of glasses of wine is okay) enters the bloodstream, the concentration of water in the blood is vastly decreased. To equalize the concentration, water goes from the skin cells into the blood, resulting in dehydrated skin cells. Because, over time, water-starved cells die, the cumulative effects of this dehydration process can add years to your looks.

In addition, alcohol depletes your body's surplus of vitamins B and C, both needed for skin health; it slows circulation (the reason alcoholics have pasty white complexions); it tends to make people eat less—or eat the wrong foods—and therefore is conducive to poor nutrition, which shows up in the skin; and, of course, it damages the liver, which is responsible for breaking down toxic substances so they don't accumulate in your body and effect unhealthy-looking skin.

Growing Intolerance to Cold Dry Air

While young skin tolerates temperature changes easily, older skin does not (especially warm to cold—I'm sure you've noticed that as soon as you hit cold dry air, your skin tends to chap and dry out much more easily than it used to). What to do: Start wearing a good rich protective cream before you head outdoors, keep a humidifier going in your home and office all the time and drink lots of water.

Another point: Older skin takes twice as long to heal as younger skin (a consideration if you're thinking of undergoing any treatment that requires healing time).

WHY SKIN GETS SAGGY, MORE WRINKLY

Breakdown of Collagen and Elastin Fibers

I'm sure you can remember when you used to wake up in the morning looking just as good, if not better, than you did before you went to sleep. Now you probably wake up with creases from scrunching your face against your pillow or your hand (see p. 31 about how to ensure yourself a wrinkle-free sleep). The reason, quite simply, is that as you age, the collagen and elastin fibers that give your skin support, resiliency and elasticity break down.

One of the primary causes of this breakdown is prolonged exposure to the sun. There's been a lot of research in the past couple of years into the sun's effect on skin, and I've devoted Chapter 7 to just that: all the latest information on how to keep your skin young-looking in spite of the sun. (Yes, you can be out in the sun without damaging your skin! And yes, you can tan healthfully!)

Other important preventive measures include key foods, vitamins and minerals (see p. 130) that help prevent wrinkles and skin-improving aerobic exercise (see p. 29).

Gravity

Believe it or not, the gravity that keeps you "down to earth" also pulls down the skin on your face, making it sag around the jaw and chin. To counteract

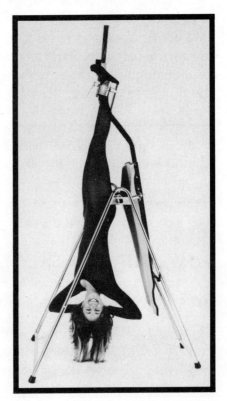

gravity, try 15 seconds to 5 minutes of inversion exercises. This is the modern term for the head and shoulder "balances" (hanging upside down) yogis have been practicing for centuries. New equipment such as The Gravity Guidance System shown opposite has made it available to the most inexperienced exerciser. Its benefits are multiple: By "inverting" the unrelenting pull of gravity, it reverses blood flow in your body, diverting it from the limbs to the brain, eyes, ears and facial skin, thus improving the look and health of your skin. It also has a stimulating effect on the lymph system, which is, in part, responsible for nourishing skin cells and eliminating their wastes; it tightens abdominals, eliminates tension and improves posture. *Warning:* Get expert help before using gravity boots; if you use them incorrectly, you could hurt yourself.

Note: If you don't have inversion boots, try 10 minutes of lying down on a slant board, or a 2-minute headstand. Or try this hip bend: Stand with feet a few inches apart and parallel, knees slightly relaxed. Bend at the hips so head and arms are hanging. Straighten knees slowly. Hold for one minute (longer if you can). Practice until your upper body goes lower as your legs straighten.

Poor Posture

When you slump you actually exacerbate the downward pull of gravity. Plus, regardless of your age, poor posture in and of itself actually makes skin look as if it's saggy. Fortunately, though, poor posture is one wrinkler you can remedy in a matter of minutes. Try this posture primer: Stand with heels two inches from a wall; head, shoulders, elbows and buttocks against the wall; hands on hips. Bend knees slightly and tighten abdominals as you tilt your pelvis so that the small of your back flattens against the wall. Tilt it back and forth ten times until you get the feel of a posture-perfect back. Then, to strengthen it, tilt pelvis and bend your knees more; rise up and down ten times, keeping your upper body pressed against the wall. Repeat two to three times daily.

Osteoporosis

You'll lose about 50 percent of your bone mass in your adult life due to osteoporosis (the gradual thinning and increasing porosity of bones, which can be accelerated by many factors). As your skull shrinks, your skin does not, and your face ends up with a lot of excess flab (see Chapter 9 for your options on nonsurgical face-lifts).

Deterioration of Teeth and Gums

Your teeth age with you: They actually become shorter, shortening the vertical dimensions of your face and often resulting in the drooping of the outer corners of the mouth, wrinkling around both top and bottom lips. See page 212 for the latest advances in cosmetic dentistry and what they can do for you.

Repeated Weight Loss and Gain

Think of a deflated balloon: That's exactly how your face will look if you lose weight too fast. *Never lose more than two pounds a week!* And never allow yourself to gain (and eventually lose) more than a total of ten pounds. Although a few pounds won't really age your skin, more will. With each weight gain, your skin will stretch to accommodate the fat. Then, when you lose it (especially if you lose it too fast), the skin will eventually sag (as it does with osteoporosis). The effects of subsequent weight gain and weight loss are cumulative.

Loss of Subcutaneous Fat

Good news: You'll lose fat with age. But don't get too excited; this is a double-edged sword. The bad news is that without its fat cushion, which contains some support fibers in addition to giving skin support of its own, your face will sag. (Loss of subcutaneous fat is usually the reason for double chins.) Is it true, then, that thin people will wrinkle more severely than fat people? Sad but true (there's some justice in the world). Coming up on page 199: the details on chemical peels, which help tighten sagging skin.

Worsening of PMS Symptoms

As you get older, you'll probably find that the symptoms of PMS (premenstrual syndrome) will either catch up with you if you never experienced them before and always wondered what all the commotion was about, or they'll worsen. One factor in particular—bloating—can leave you with what I call fat wrinkles as well as undereye bags. The causes are twofold: First, in PMS there's an imbalance of estrogen and progesterone levels, which leads to the fluid retention that causes swelling in the face (and body). And second, there are excess secretions of the pituitary hormone ACTH, which compounds the problem.

What you can do: Susan M. Lark, M.D., director of the PMS Self Help Center in Los Altos, California, and author of *Susan Lark's Premenstrual Syndrome Self-Help Book*, told me you can beat the problem by eating antibloating foods: very lean protein (fish and poultry); foods high in vitamin B_6 like salmon, tuna, beans and whole grains; and bitter greens like watercress, escarole and dandelion leaves.

THE PERFECT ANTIBLOAT DINNER:
Broiled fish or chicken, brown rice, bitter greens mixed salad, and herb tea.

To avoid bloating, omit the following foods from your diet when possible:

- Salt (instead use a potassium-based salt substitute like Morton's powder that comes in salt-shaker form; or light soy sauce—$1/4$ teaspoon = 1 teaspoon salt).
- Sugar (instead of table sugar use maple syrup, honey, unsweetened apple juice; substitute sugar in recipes, too—$3/4$ cup sugar = $1/2$ cup honey, $1/4$ cup molasses, $1/2$ cup maple syrup).
- High-fat foods (try goat or sheep cheese instead of cheeses made from cow's milk; soy and nut milks, available at health food stores, instead of whole milk . . . and stay away from processed foods).

Also, be sure you're getting enough vitamin B_6 (take a supplement and try some easy yoga exercises such as the plow on page 28) when you're feeling particularly bloated.

Smoking and Smokers' Smoke: Real Skin Hazards

I began smoking when I was fourteen—one cigarette at a time in the bath-room—and was easily working my way through three packs a day by my

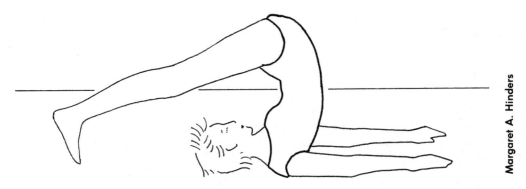

The plow

early thirties. I felt great, and since I was no jock I never detected any deterioration of my stamina. I had no intention of quitting until I started dating the man who is now my husband.

Unlike me, Benjamin is a jock and a fitness fanatic. He hated my smoking, and I honestly think that had I not quit, he wouldn't have married me. To please him, I decided to go to the Schick Center for Control of Smoking in Los Angeles, California, and try to give it up.

My first session was a disaster—at least in the counselors' eyes. It's their job to motivate people into quitting. They presented me with all the hard facts on related illnesses, all to no avail. It was bad, but not bad enough or scary enough to get me to stop.

What finally worked: a very clever counselor found my weak spot—vanity. He explained how smoking instantly adds ten years to your looks. That was it for me. I quit then and there. That was eight years ago and I haven't had a cigarette since!

My point is not to gloat but to try to convince you, too, to stop smoking—and thus stop wrinkling—because it's now thought that the smoker's skin wrinkles up to ten years sooner than that of nonsmokers, depending on the duration and intensity of the habit. Here's why smoking is harmful to your skin: (1) Nicotine constricts blood vessels, reducing the flow of blood that brings nourishment to skin cells and eliminates their impurities, too. (2) Cigarettes can destroy your body's supply of skin-saving vitamin C, essential in the formation of collagen as well as of oxygen-carrying red blood cells. If your skin cells aren't properly oxygenated they "suffocate," taking on a gray-

Margaret A. Hinders

ish cast. Most nutritionists recommend that smokers take vitamin C supplements at the rate of 25 milligrams per cigarette. (3) The simple act of grasping cigarette upon cigarette with the lips and inhaling results in fine lines on the upper lip.

> The bad news for noncigarette smokers: Just being in a smoke-filled room can cause skin damage. The reason is that the smoke particles stay suspended in the air as though they were pollution, and you breathe in a large fraction of those particles.

Smog/Pollution

If you live in a city you are more prone to wrinkling than rural dwellers, because the major pollutants you breathe in—mainly ozone and nitrogen dioxide—produce a toxic effect that is extremely aging to your skin. Studies have shown that by taking daily supplements of 8 mg of vitamin E, you can alleviate—in fact, negate!—city wrinkles.

WHY SKIN LOSES ITS YOUTHFUL GLOW

Circulation Slowdown

With age, the blood supply that flows to the skin, nourishing it with nutrients and oxygen, diminishes—and you lose your naturally rosy cheeks and general healthy youthful look.

To the rescue: regular aerobic exercise. Here's why.

- Exercise boosts blood circulation, which, in turn, ups the rate at which skin cells receive oxygen and nutrients. The flush on your face after a good workout is a sign that your skin has just had a real meal.
- Exercise gradually increases blood volume; that means more nutrients and more oxygen are carried to the skin.

And, in addition . . .

- *Exercise precipitates perspiration, which flushes out dirt and impurities, such as uric acid, from the skin and brings more natural moisturizers to the epidermis.*
- *Exercise raises skin temperature—from 86° F. to 98.6° F.—and in doing so steps up the production of collagen, which keeps skin thick and young-looking.*
- *Exercise may make it easier for you to quit skin-damaging smoking, according to several recent studies.*
- *Exercise can relieve stress,* which shows up eventually as lines on the face. A fit person produces less of the so-called stress-producing hormones called catecholamines; more serotonin, a muscle relaxant chemically similar to a tranquillizer; and more betaendorphine, which produces feelings of calm and optimism.
- *Exercise burns calories and will help you maintain your weight and avoid the yo-yo syndrome of repeated weight gains and losses, which age skin dramatically.* I recommend 30 to 60 minutes of exercise a day, five to six days a week: That means you'll burn 300 to 600 calories a day; if you cut out 300 calories a day, you could realize up to a 600-calorie deficit a day, or 3,600 calories a week. Since a pound is equal to 3,500 calories, that's a pound a week (a healthy rate that'll allow you to keep the weight off and keep your skin taut and resilient, too).

Cell-shedding Slowdown

Another reason you lose your youthful glow and, perhaps, gain an uneven skin tone, too: The dead cells at the top of your epidermis are not being shed as effectively or as fast as they used to be. While young skin naturally gets rid of these cells and replaces them with fresh new cells within fifteen to twenty days, older skin requires twenty-five to thirty-five days for the same process. In plain language, what this means is that the dead cells remain on the surface of your skin too long; they clump together, clogging pores and causing an ashen, sometimes leathery look. Thus the absolute importance of stepping up your exfoliating as you get older. More about that in Chapter 3, too.

Reduction of Melanin Production

One final reason for the loss of your youthful glow: Your skin stops producing as many melanocytes, which produce melanin, the substance that gives your skin most of its color. Not only does your ability to tan decrease (later you'll learn why a light tan is one of your best protectors from the sun's harmful rays), but there is also a visible lightening of skin tone. Plus, an uneven distribution of these melanocytes may result in uneven skintone or, in the case of too many in one spot, the appearance of the brown frecklelike splotches sometimes referred to as liver spots (but obviously having nothing to do with the liver) that most frequently turn up on your hands.

You can, of course, use makeup to cover uneven skin tones. Exfoliation can help slough away unevenness. As for removal of liver spots, see page 50; and see page 51 for the facts on cryosurgery and mild chemical peeling.

HOW TO HAVE A WRINKLE-FREE SLEEP . . . SO YOU CAN WAKE UP (AND STAY) YOUNGER-LOOKING

You may think that while you sleep, your skin is free from potential wrinklers, but it isn't. In fact, during sleep, skin is quite vulnerable to aging for several reasons: It's now that skin works harder, regenerating, metabolizing nutrients and eliminating wastes at its peak rates. So what you do—and don't do— for your skin while you sleep can have a profound effect on how you look the next morning . . . and in years to come.

The three main factors that age your skin at night:

- fluid retention
- creasing
- dryness

Fluid Retention

When you're in a prone position, your body fluids tend to collect in facial tissues, making you wake with a puffy face and especially puffy eyes (the reason that too much sleep can sometimes make you look more tired than too little). What can help: raising the bed head with books wedged between the mattress and box spring and/or elevating your head and feet on a pillow to improve circulation; cut down on salt and alcohol, too.

Creasing

There are two reasons you probably awaken with sleep creases now: first, if you've been scrunching your face into a pillow or your hand for eight hours, and, second, if you've been "expressing" yourself during sleep (i.e., you grind your teeth due to stress, or you squint). In both cases the wrinkles are temporary (they'll fade within a couple hours of rising), but after awakening day after day, year after year with sleep creases, it's not unlikely that they'll become permanent fixtures. What to do?

1. *Sleep face up.* When Catherine was at *Bazaar* she interviewed a famous model who said that her only means of compensating for years of sun damage was to train herself to sleep face up. Though it was difficult

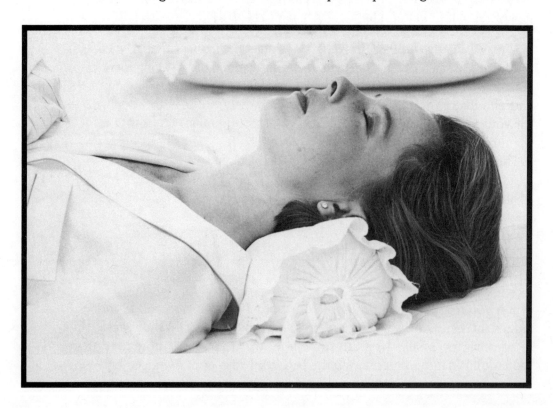

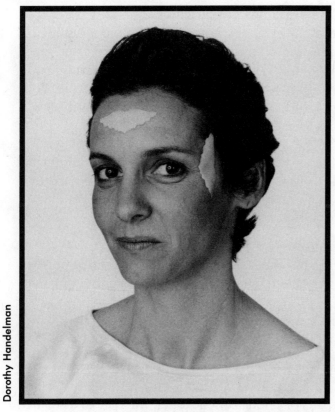

Dorothy Handelman

Wings

at first, she managed, and now she literally always sleeps that way as a matter of habit. If you've tried and failed, train yourself to sleep with your face slightly away from the pillow, which should be a small flat baby pillow under the nape of your neck.

2. *Make sure your bedroom has good shades and/or get an eye mask.* Another model told Catherine that when she travels she takes an eye mask just in case there are no shades. "It seems such a waste to squint and cause wrinkles while you sleep!"

3. *Stop expressing yourself at night.* If you express yourself during sleep—most commonly by grinding teeth or frowning (thereby wrinkling your forehead in response to tension)—find a way to stop. Drink a glass of warm milk, take a hot bath, put on some soothing music—anything to relax before going to bed. One more thought: You can apply adhesive-backed Wings anywhere you don't want lines to form at night (forehead, laugh lines or crow's feet). You simply massage

your wrinkles for a few seconds, splash them with cold water to stimulate circulation in the area, dry your skin and place moistened Wings over them, pressing until they stick firmly. Every time you express yourself, you'll feel it! After at least 15 minutes (overnight, if possible), remove Wings gently by moistening with warm water. To order, write to Wings Products Co. Inc., Box 680, East Hampton, New York 11937 (50 Wings/$4.25 plus 75¢ shipping).

Should you awaken with sleep creases and can't wait the two hours it takes for them to fade naturally, here's a routine I developed that erases them almost on the spot.

- First, *cleanse.*
- Then, *slather on moisturizer*—be generous.
- Next, *bathe, or shower* in hot water (the steam plumps up fine lines) or apply warm water, washcloth and compresses to your face for five minutes.
- *Blot off* remaining moisturizer with a tissue.
- Finally, *rinse* with cold water.

Or try this shock treatment I learned from Diane Young (Diane Young Skin Care Center, New York City): Brew chamomile tea with mineral water; cool and mix with equal parts of a nonalcoholic toner. Add half of a crushed vitamin B_6 tablet. Mix well and freeze in a plastic ice cube tray, filling each cube half-full and angling in a tongue depressor (available in pharmacies). In the A.M., when you want to wake up your face and smooth away sleep creases, pop out one cube and use the stick as a handle to rub over your face. (See opposite.) Pat dry. Moisturize and apply makeup as usual.

Dryness

Unless your bedroom is in the middle of a rain forest, you'd do well to be aware of your skin's water loss—due to heat or air conditioning—during sleep. This is one reason it's so important to cleanse and apply night creams before bed and to turn on a humidifier. You don't want to drink too many fluids before bed because too many fluids can exacerbate the flow of fluids to the face and cause puffiness. Another possible irritant: the drying detergents used to launder linens. Try switching detergents.

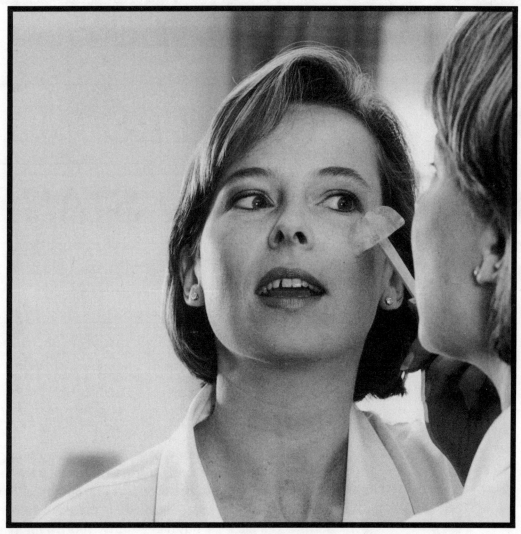

Shock treatment

If this chapter full of skin agers seems hopelessly long, take heart. No matter what the reasons for your wrinkling, there's a surprising amount you can do—from proper skin care and makeup application to nonsurgical face-lifts—to prevent further aging, even turn back the hands of time to look younger! Coming up: everything you need to know to do just that, plus a complete resource list (Chapter 10) of whom to go to for what.

TWO

THE AGE GAUGES:

WHERE WRINKLES

BEGIN, WHAT TO START

DOING...NOW

Wrinkles seem to turn up overnight. One morning you wake up and suddenly they're there—at least that's how it happens to most women. But in reality aging is a natural process that starts the day you're born, accelerates slightly after thirty, more rapidly thereafter. To help you determine whether your skin is starting to show signs of aging, here are some questions to ask yourself. One yes and, yes, you'll just have to face the fact that your skin is beginning to show its years.

- Does your skin look paler?
- Do people say you look tired even when you're not?

- Have you been accused of looking unhappy, sullen, pouty—even though you're not?
- Does your foundation (the one you've been wearing for years) suddenly look like a mask?
- Is your skin more sensitive? Does it react more strongly and visibly to, say, temperature changes?
- Do your cheeks look and feel more hollow?
- When you pinch the skin under your cheekbones, does it feel flabby?
- When you put your hands on your jawline, do you feel some excess flesh that wasn't always there?

So that you can be aware of what to expect and when to expect it, I've put together a very general guide to the age ranges and stages of aging. Remember, they're broad; there are numerous factors—say, how much time you spend in the sun, how diligent you've been about sticking to a well-balanced diet and exercise routine, how hectic your life is and how well you've learned to contain your stress levels—that can affect the aging process. If, for example, you've been prudent with your skin-care regimen, your wrinkles may appear later than this guide indicates; if not, they may turn up at a younger age. The bottom line, though, is simple and universal: You will wrinkle at some point.

If this sounds depressing (and I have to admit it does), don't despair. As sure as wrinkles are a fact of life, so it is absolutely true that modern technology (advances in skin-care products and treatments, state-of-the-art makeup products and application techniques, as well as new hairstyling products and coloring and perming techniques) will help you look better for your age than ever before. And you can do so with less effort.

I want to reiterate that your goal should be to look your optimum best for your current age. In my mind, a woman who tries to look years younger is trying to change who she is; a woman who is uncomfortable with herself is not attractive whether she's under twenty or over sixty. What I do find attractive is a woman who's thirty-five, forty-five, fifty-five, sixty-five or older, looks it and feels great about it.

Anyway, there are a few places, such as your eyes, neck and hands, that will reveal your age no matter what you do. Here's exactly what you can expect . . . exactly when.

Ages	Stages
16–24	Teenage oiliness begins to clear, signaling a slowing (albeit a visually imperceptible one) of oil-gland production.
25–30	Oil production slows perceptibly and skin starts to show signs of dryness—if not all over then in distinct patches, especially near the hairline. If skin is thin and delicate, laugh lines around the mouth and the outer corner of eyes will start to turn up.
31–35	Skin thins markedly, especially around eyes and mouth. Squint lines form at the corners of eyes. Frown lines appear on the forehead.
36–40	You will notice that your skin is losing its elasticity: Eyelids will get heavier; lines around eyes, on the forehead and mouth will deepen; and neck skin will begin to sag. You may see, too, the beginnings of an unevenness in your skin tone.
41–50	Fine lines will deepen to form wrinkles around your eyes and mouth and on your forehead. Eyelids will become droopy and crepey-looking; vertical lines will form on your upper lip, and laugh lines around mouth and eyes as well as forehead furrows will become more prominent. Your cheeks will begin to look hollow as skin thins and loses its tautness all the way to the base of the neck. (A double chin may start to form, too.) Skin tone will dull, become pale.
50–on	Expect the wrinkles around eyes and mouth and on the forehead to become even deeper, bags to form under the eyes. There will be a conspicuous dropping of the lower half of your face—more flesh along the jawline, a definite double chin and folds in neck skin. The tip of the nose and the earlobes will drop. Your color will become paler and rougher in texture. Expect, too, broken capillaries and brown spots (and wrinkles) on hands (and sometimes on the face, too). The risk of skin cancer is double at 70 what it is at 30.

WRINKLE-FREE EYES

They're a dead giveaway: The most expressive part of your face, your eyes are the first thing people see when they meet you. The skin around the eyes is thinner and contains fewer oil and sweat glands to keep it moist and smooth than does the skin on the rest of your face. Therefore, it's destined to be among the first areas to lose elasticity and resiliency. Plus, laughing, crying—

even your hands on your face—move the skin around your eyes. It's no wonder that crow's-feet and undereye lines develop early on and that your lids eventually droop and stretch out of shape.

Sad, and too true. But equally realistic: There's lots you can do—easily! simply!—to get rid of eye lines. Makeup is the most obvious way, and I've devoted a whole chapter to makeup tips and tricks (see Chapter 4). Looking for a more permanent solution? You can choose among different nonsurgical lifts (all of this coming up in Chapter 9). Diet can help, too (see Chapter 6), and so can proper skin care (see Chapter 3). Right here, though, are some very specific solutions to eye lines culled from the experts as well as from friends. They've worked for me; maybe some will help you, too.

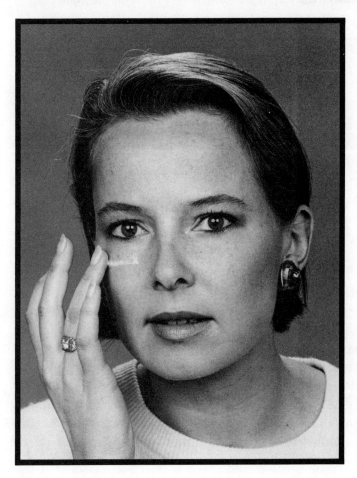

Dab on, don't rub in eye cream

Moisturizing

A lot of women use a moisturizer on their faces but forget their eyes. Don't! To apply: Very gently dab cream on from the outside of your eye toward your nose, concentrating on the skin under the eye (not too close to lashes! You'll find that it'll migrate upward naturally) and on the outside corner where crow's-feet tend to develop.

Travel tip: Once I forgot to pack my eye cream when I was on a business trip, and I found that my lip moisturizer worked beautifully as a night treatment because of its emollient waxy consistency. It's too greasy for daytime use, however.

Making Up

It's absolutely imperative that you apply your makeup with a light hand. A sable brush or cotton Q-Tip applicator will simplify putting on shadows gently. If you use your fingers, you'll use too much pressure on the delicate skin. I try to avoid using hard eyeliner pencils, which always seem to pull my skin as I draw the line, and if I must use one, I just make sure the point of the eye pencil is super sharp and also very soft. Catherine rubs the point of any pencil she uses on her eyes with a tissue to soften it.

When applying shadows, liners and mascara, do so looking down into a mirror to keep you from opening your eyes wide and wrinkling your forehead (as most women do). This may not sound like a big deal, but consider this: *Putting on eye makeup at least once, probably twice, a day in a manner that causes habitual wrinkling can be very damaging (aging!) indeed.* (See opposite.)

A few notes on mascara. First, discard it every two months; because of its consistency, it tends to contaminate faster than other cosmetics. Second, use the most fiber-free formulation you can find and apply it thoroughly, but don't overdo—you don't want fibers or mascara flakes to work their way into the eye, causing redness and irritation. Third, be careful not to let mascara smear onto the lids (apply carefully); it's fine for lashes, too drying for lid skin.

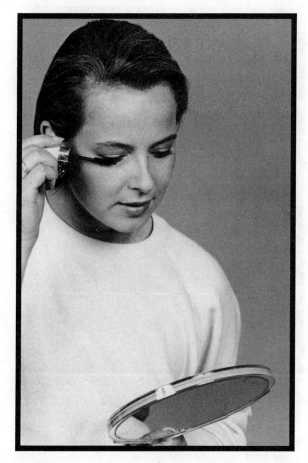

Putting on mascara

The Only Way to Remove Eye Makeup

Just as it's imperative to be gentle when you moisturize eyes or apply makeup, it's equally crucial to remove eye makeup carefully or you'll create premature lines. I recommend using a special eye makeup remover, not an ordinary cleanser, which doesn't do the job as easily and will incite rubbing, and cotton, not tissue, which has microscopic splintery fibers in it that can irritate delicate skin around the eye. I like oil-based removers; Catherine prefers the oil-free variety because she says the oilier ones never fail to seep into her eyes and onto her contacts. We both use the large-size cotton puffs, the kind

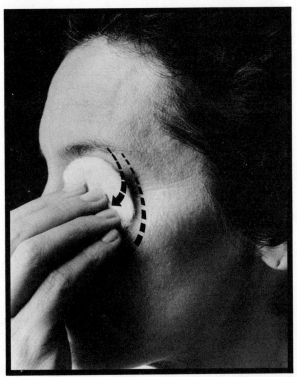

Dorothy Handelman

that come in bags of a hundred, and prefer them to the flat cotton pads, which aren't as soft.

To remove makeup: Saturate the cotton with the remover. Close the eye you're going to cleanse and, counting to 5, gently press the cotton against the eye, moving it from the eyebrow, over the lid and down over lashes. This will prevent the remover from getting into your eyes and will allow the makeup to dissolve into the lotion so it won't require rubbing. *Never rub!* Also, downward rather than horizontal strokes will prevent lash fallout. Continue with more cotton and more remover until all traces of makeup are gone. Splash with cold water.

Easy Eye Youtheners

Fatigue, irritation, swelling—they all age eyes, making you look older and more haggard than you really are. Here is how to refresh tired, sensitive and/or puffy eyes

Try rebounding—Rebounding is exercising to music (or not) by jumping, turning, twisting, dancing, jogging, or doing calisthenics on a nylon-floored cousin of the trampoline (it's only 3 to 4 feet in size, only 6 to 7 inches from the floor). It's so much fun that it keeps participants coming back far more regularly over longer periods of time than any other form of exercise. Bonus: Women using rebounding to lose weight and get in shape also get rid of bags under their eyes, according to James R. White, Ph.D., director of the Exercise Physiology and Rehabilitation Lab in the Department of Physical Education at the University of California at San Diego.

Quick eye wash—Bathe eyes in cold water or witch hazel; you'll reduce puffiness within a half-hour or so.

Compresses (best used with 4-inch-wide cotton or individual cotton pads while you're lying down, for 15 to 20 minutes, feet elevated on a pillow)—Try milk (the lactic acid has healing power) or raw potato slices (between two pieces of cotton on lids).

Preventive measures—Don't wear makeup for a few days if eyes are puffy—irritation could be caused by sensitivity to one of the products • If you wake up with puffy eyes, you may be using too heavy an eye cream and applying too much too close to the eyes. Go for less, of a lighter variety • Check your

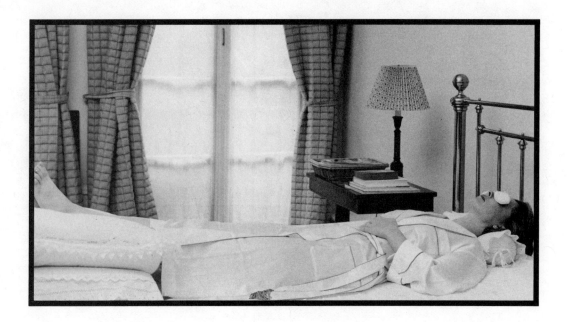

eye makeup removal routine—it could be too vigorous • Switch from a waterproof mascara (which is harder to remove than nonwaterproof ones and requires a potentially irritating oily remover) and from sparkly to matte makeup (iridescents often require a lot of rubbing to remove completely) • Sleep with your head elevated and try not to drink too many fluids, particularly alcohol, right before bedtime • Reduced salt intake can eliminate puffiness • Every night before bed get into the habit of doing the following undereye smoother, which will decongest the water and fatty deposits that can form bags: For 5 seconds, press against the bridge of your nose next to inside corners of your eyes with the softest part of the pads of your index fingers. Move fingers down to the base of eye socket and press here for 5 seconds. Then move them outward along the socket bone, stopping to press firmly at random points for 5 seconds until you reach past the temple to the hairline.

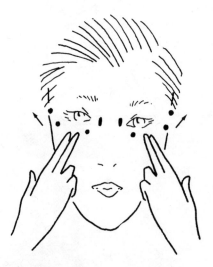

Margaret A. Hinders

Vitamins for young eyes—Though I have my Antiwrinkle Vitamin and Mineral Plan coming up, I want to note right here the two vitamins that are especially helpful in keeping the skin around eyes healthy and young-looking.

• *Vitamin C* (found in citrus fruits, green and yellow vegetables). Vitamin C is necessary for strong capillary walls and connective tissue. Since it is not stored in the body and must be replenished daily, it may be a good idea to take a vitamin C supplement every day (250 mg.) if you notice fine lines forming around the eyes. And stop smoking: Smoking robs your system of vitamin C and tends to make you squint, too!

· *Vitamin B complex* (found in green and yellow vegetables, whole grains, brewer's yeast, yogurt). A deficiency in B complex can not only cause deterioration of the myelin sheath that surrounds the eyes' optic nerve pathways but also the deterioration of the youthful look of the skin around eyes. See page 134 for the proper supplement dosage.

A YOUNGER-LOOKING NECK

Be aware of your neck, and beware of wrinkling there. Like your eyes, your neck has thin skin, with less oil and sweat glands than the rest of your body. It has less of a fatty layer, too, which can give skin a plump, youthful appearance. In addition, poor posture (if you have a tendency to slump and stand round-shouldered) will weaken the neck muscles and, in turn, contribute to wrinkling and, perhaps, a double chin.

Just for kicks, *don't move:* Feel your neck in whatever position you're reading this. Now put the book down, stand up straight and hold your head high, as if it were being pulled up by an invisible string attached from the top of your head. Drop your shoulders, look ahead and feel your neck. Does it feel longer, firmer, smoother? Get the idea?

You should treat your neck as if it's an extension of your face: Cleanse it with facial cleanser (not a body soap, which can be dehydrating and harsh); use an alcohol-free toner to tighten pores and keep them taut (I like to mix my toner with equal parts cold water and spray it on my neck with a plant mister); and apply a moisturizer every time you apply one to your face. Don't forget sun screen either!

The right exercise can help guard against wrinkling, too. Try this neck stretch (it helps release tension that collects in the neck): Sit with legs straight out in front of you, feet flexed and about 6 inches apart, hands clasped behind head, elbows back. Inhale as you lift your torso. Exhale, round your back and bend to touch chin to chest (let elbows relax and come closer together). Inhale, return to starting position. Repeat five times slowly.

Here are two more good ones. First, a neck firmer: Without clenching your teeth, smile as wide as you can (as if you were making an "eeeck" sound), tensing the muscles in your neck and jaw. Relax. Repeat several times

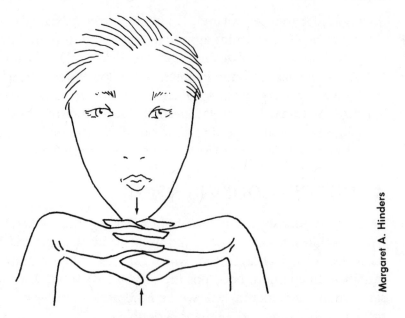

Margaret A. Hinders

for 1 minute. Second, an isometric muscle strengthener (do it at least once a day): Sit with elbows on a table, chin on folded interlaced fingers. Press down with your chin as you press up with your fists. Hold for 20 seconds, relax, and repeat twenty times.

HAND DE-AGERS

Next to your eyes and your neck, your hands can be your biggest age traitors. I'm sure you've seen plenty of women with firm, relatively unlined faces— and hands that are dry and wrinkled. The skin on hands (like that around eyes and on your neck) is extremely thin; just take a minute to feel how tightly stretched it is. It also contains relatively few oil and sweat glands. Combine this with more facts: first, that your hands take a daily beating as you expose them to extreme temperatures (say, in cold air and hot water); second, that you use them a lot; and third, that you often forget to care for them. Think about it: Every time you put on moisturizer, do you slather your hands with a lubricating lotion, too? And every time you put a sun screen on your face, do you put a sun screen on your hands, too?

Here is everything you need to know about caring for—and de-aging— your hands.

Moisturizing

- Many hand models have told me that their secret is vitamin E oil; they say it keeps their hands smooth and moist (plus it heals cuts and irritations overnight).

- Once a week give your hands a facial (it's much easier—and less time consuming—than a manicure because you don't have to worry about smudging polish). Here's how, from skin-care expert Aida Grey: Apply a moisturizing face mask to fingers and top of hands up to your wrist; let it dry and then wash off with lukewarm water. Follow by slathering on a rich, emollient hand moisturizer/cream, especially on skin around the cuticles (if you don't have a good one, just use your facial moisturizer or, better yet, your night cream—or soak hands in olive oil as hot as is comfortable for ten minutes. Blot off excess with a tissue). Then put on cotton gloves (you can get inexpensive ones at the dime store). If you can sleep like this, great; if not, remove them in an hour. I guarantee you'll see a difference immediately!

- Great news for hands that tend to dry out and crack in winter (cold weather is a killer for hands: Lack of moisture in the air outside and

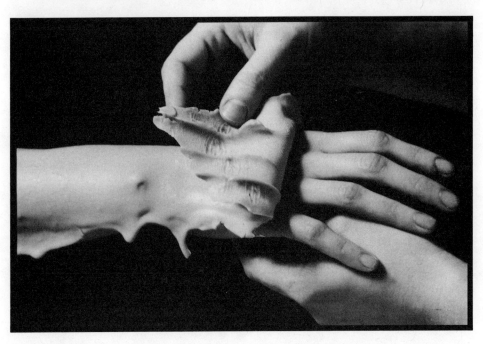

dry steam heat inside combine to damage the natural moisture barrier that protects hands from drying out). Hydrocortisone cream that is sold over the counter is a super healer!

- The same lack of moisture that dries out your hands in winter also affects your nails and cuticles, which, though they have nothing to do with wrinkles, can contribute to making hands look unattractive and older than they are. Keep a cuticle cream next to your bed and rub in a small amount before you turn out the light.
- Whatever moisturizer you choose to use on your hands, keep it readily available or you'll never use it. Keep a small tube of hand cream in your bathroom and near the kitchen sink. At work, leave a large bottle in the bathroom (one in your desk drawer, too). Enlist your colleagues into taking turns replenishing the supply. Tip (learned through personal experience): Choose something inexpensive so people aren't tempted to take it home with them.
- Also super healing: *milk*. Simply soak hands in a bowl of warm milk for 10 minutes, rinse and moisturize.

Cleansing

- Get in the habit of using lukewarm rather than hot water to wash your hands—it's much less drying.
- Recently I started using a scented body cleanser to wash my hands— they feel great afterward and they smell like the rest of me, too.
- During the cold weather months make sure you wash your hands with only a mild soap. In fact, if your hands are really chapped and cracked, it's a good idea to use the same cleanser (moisturizer, too) you use on your face.
- After washing your hands, don't dry them completely . . . and apply a moisturizer (it'll lock in the water).

Manicuring

I, for one, have never had beautifully manicured hands on a consistent basis. I can neither get to the manicurist regularly nor do I have the discipline to give myself a manicure. Nonetheless, I realize manicures are well worth the time and/or money—they make hands look younger—and, from the constant care, they make women aware of their hands and nails. So here's my new solution: I've now started having my manicurist come to my home. It's not that much more expensive and it's an incredible luxury. A lot of manicurists like to do at-home manicures to make some extra money; ask yours the next time you see her.

Here's a *nail color guide* that makes wrinkled hands look less wrinkled. Choose according to your skin color (hold bottles against your skin to see which is best).

For fair skin types: red and orange colors.

For ruddy complexions: blue-reds.

For olive and black skins: pink-reds, pink-corals.

When skin has a translucent quality: mauves, plums.

To avoid, no matter what your coloring: deep purples and maroons—they make skin look sallow, accent lines, too.

Protection

I know you've heard this a million times . . . but, in order to protect your hands from too much hot water and irritating detergents, rubber gloves are a must. I could never force myself to put on rubber gloves because they were so uncomfortable and they never fit right. When I was interviewing a manicurist for a story we were doing in *Bazaar*, I got the perfect solution: surgical gloves, which are so thin and fit so tightly they're like wearing a second skin. They're great, and I really do use them. And for added protection, I apply hand cream before putting on the gloves (the cream also makes it easier to slip into them). You can find these gloves at any pharmacy or surgical supply house, and they're pretty cheap, too.

You also should protect your hands from the sun with a sun screen (SPF 15 or higher) when you're outdoors. This doesn't mean just when you're basking in the sun, either, but when you're gardening, playing golf or tennis or just taking a walk. For sports, when you want dry, not greasy, palms, apply an oil-free sun screen formulated for oily skin. And remember: Every time you wash your hands, swim or dry the perspiration off them, you need to reapply the sun screen. Plus, get in the daily habit of wearing a hand cream that contains a sun screen.

Here's a treatment Catherine and I use before we go out at night: Wet hands and don't dry them completely. Mix a hand lotion with a few drops of foundation (or use one of the new tinted moisturizers for the face). Apply to hands, blending well. It'll give you a nice smooth look and cover imperfections, too.

Camouflaging Brown Spots

Whether you've taken care of your hands or not, by the time you're in your forties you may notice the appearance of brown, frecklelike spots (liver spots) on the backs of your hands and wrists (often, too, on your forehead, cheeks or upper lip). Caused by the slowing of the cell renewal rate that is basic to aging, the spots most commonly turn up when skin cells divide so gradually they pick up melanin from nearby pigment-producing cells. They're sometimes, too, produced by the interaction of the sun on skin in combination with another ingredient—often bergamot, a substance found in some fragrances. Some nutritionists claim a good B complex vitamin is all it takes to clear up brown spots, but if this doesn't work for you, you have several other options.

- If you want an easy, painless and inexpensive solution, I'd try one of the many bleaching creams specifically designed to make brown spots disappear. Available over the counter, these creams work on pigment problems in the upper layers of the skin by preventing production of new pigment in the spotted area, which, in time, just sloughs off (the creams don't actually fade the area). You should see results in two months. Or make your own bleaching cream by combining enough salt and lemon juice (or vinegar) to make a paste; leave on for about 30 minutes.
- Have you tried the creams but found they don't work? This is probably because your dark spots emanate from layers of skin too deep to slough

off with over-the-counter creams. See a dermatologist, who can prescribe a cream with a higher concentration of the "bleaching" agent hydroquinone.

· If this prescription cream doesn't help the problem, your dermatologist might recommend cryosurgery or a mild chemical peel. These methods offer the advantage of speed, and the spots are guaranteed not to return unless you expose your hands to the sun without the protection of sun screen. *If your hands aren't terribly wrinkled but do have brown spots, I'd go with cryosurgery.* A very cold liquid nitrogen is applied directly on the spot and destroys the cells; the spot peels off (on the spot!), and you are left without any sign of the spot ever being there. *If your hands are wrinkled and have brown spots, your best bet is a mild chemical peel.* The procedure is like the one used on the face (see p. 199). The chemical is applied not just to the spot but to the entire tops of the hands, producing a controlled burn much like a sunburn. The skin responds by shedding its top layer and replacing it with a new layer of skin that is younger-looking, smoother and wrinkle-free. Healing time is three to five days.

EXPRESSION IMPRESSIONS

You should be aware that there is one age gauge that shows up on some people and not others, and earlier on some than on others: expression lines.

Expression lines are wrinkles you cause yourself by regular moving of facial muscles. Women, more naturally expressive than men, use their facial muscles more frequently and, because women's skin is thinner than men's, the lines these expressions cause are deeper. (And, unfortunately, while men's expression lines are considered to give them character, the lines women get are considered signs of age.)

This is not to say that you should stop smiling or being yourself. But every smile, every frown, every pursed lip eventually, if done continually over time, leaves an impression on your face—first in fine lines, then later as wrinkles. What I do suggest is that you become conscious of your facial expressions, because there are certain things you can do—without sacrificing your personality—to keep them from causing wrinkles. One way to increase your awareness follows.

The Mental Face-lift

Sit in a quiet dark room, feet flat on the floor, hands resting quietly in your lap, eyes closed. Concentrate on relaxing all over. First, focus all your attention on relaxing your eyes: the brows from the outside in to the spot between them; then the eyelids and, finally, the eyes themselves. Next, eyes still closed, focus on your nose from the top to the bottom and the width of it, too, as it curves onto the plane of your cheeks. Now the mouth: Release the tension in your lips until you feel your jaw drop and relax. Drop your shoulders and let all the tension go in your neck. Drop your head forward, touch your chin to your chest, roll it to the right, then back, then to the left, breathing continuously as you go. Reverse directions and repeat each circle two more times.

FAUX WRINKLES

Do you sometimes look in the mirror, see lots of lines, panic . . . then look again the next day or sometimes even a few hours later and find they're gone? Faux wrinkles are very real when they're there, but if you know their potential causes and cures (none has to do with aging!), you can eliminate these nonpermanent lines once and for all!

It could be that you're *overcleansing and/or not moisturizing enough.* This is particularly common among women with oily skin—and they often compound the problem by overusing acne preparations. What results is parched skin, which, in turn, means fine lines. What to do: As far as acne preparations go, use them judiciously, only once a day until your skin can build up a tolerance. And change your skin care routine immediately—switch to products that treat oily skin without making it oilier or totally drying it out. Try a gentler cleanser and a good oil-free moisturizer (see p. 62 for ways to tell if your moisturizer is working). Unfortunately many women with oily skin still don't understand that they need a moisturizer—not the same rich one a person with dry skin may need but a lighter one that can work beautifully and never cause the skin to break out.

Certain medications can cause faux wrinkles, too. I've had problems with diuretics and some antibiotics. I occasionally take diuretics for PMS bloat. At first, every time I took one my skin felt tighter and drier, and lines that were never there seemed to appear immediately; the lines that were evident seemed to be deeper, too. And I know I wasn't imagining it because my husband even noticed. I finally put two and two together, and whenever I take a diuretic now, I step up my moisturizing routine—I use a product richer than my normal lightweight one and I moisturize midday as well as morning and evening. I also find that antibiotics dry and temporarily line my skin, as do sinus medications and some cold tablets. When I take them, too, I switch moisturizers—and drink lots of water.

Another cause of faux wrinkles: *a change in climate*, especially going from warm weather to a cold climate where there's less moisture in the air. Under these conditions even the oiliest skin can suffer from dehydration and fine lines. (More on this in Chapter 3.)

RED WRINKLES: BROKEN CAPILLARIES

True, they're not wrinkles per se, but broken capillaries turn up as fine red lines that do indeed reveal one's age. They're most visible in fair, thin-skinned people, most common on people in their late forties on. They occur when the walls of the blood vessels themselves start to thin and when skin has lost the elasticity required to help vessels resist normal pressure of the blood. But, as with real wrinkles, anyone can get broken capillaries at any time. Don't despair: There are precautions you can take to hold them off for a time and/or keep them from becoming as bad as they might if you took no precautions at all.

Avoid the following:

- Extreme temperatures—don't ever use ice cold or very hot water on your face.
- Extreme temperature changes—don't, for example, come in from the cold and head straight for a blazing fire.
- Too much sun in winter or in summer—don't forget sun protection and stick to the tan plan in Chapter 7.
- Alcohol—it causes red blood cells to pile up and clog blood vessels; as a result, cells don't get enough oxygen and begin to deteriorate, causing small hemorrhages or leakages in the capillaries.
- Spicy foods, coffee and tea—if your face flushes when you eat them . . . stop.

- Harsh abrasive facial scrubs (use cream-based ones) and coarse facial brushes.
- Squeezing blackheads and pimples too harshly.
- Saunas, steam and chlorine-laden pools.
- General inactivity—the more immobile you are, the more circulation slows and the more likely blood is to collect, increasing pressure on the vessels and causing them to break.

Do the following:

- Exercise.
- Stick to a balanced diet.
- Make sure you're getting plenty of vitamins (C, E, B complex) and of the mineral zinc (all helpful in assuring smooth, even circulation).
- Give yourself regular gentle facial massages (or have a professional one) to stimulate circulation.
- Keep skin well lubricated.
- Use calming, soothing products (vasoconstrictors). Vasoconstricting ingredients, which are found most commonly in facial masks, include allantoin, aloe vera, azulene, calamine, chamomile, ginseng, panthenol and rose hips.

If your broken capillaries are very bad, the best way to get rid of them is with *electrodesiccation*. A dermatologist uses a fine titanium needle and a low electric current to collapse and dissipate the vessels. The procedure is 80 percent effective after the first treatment; it is uncomfortable and/or painful, but you won't see even a trace of your red lines afterward. The bad news, though, is that people who have had broken capillaries once will probably get them again in other places.

Some doctors are using *argon lasers* to get rid of broken capillaries, but there is no advantage to using this procedure over electrodesiccation; plus it takes longer to do, with more risks.

THREE

WRINKLE REMOVING

TREATMENTS AND

PRODUCTS

It's a constant refrain from readers and friends alike: What products should I use on my skin and do they really work?

I can certainly understand the confusion, what with all the thousands of products on the market and the seemingly never-ending bombardment of advertising claims. In a nutshell, here's my position: No product can really erase wrinkles. But if you've stayed away from using them because of this, you're being very shortsighted and are actually shortchanging yourself. When they are used daily and consistently, skin-care products definitely will minimize lines and make skin look younger. Take the women we photograph for *Bazaar*—and not just the models either: Those who use treatment products religiously have better skin than those who don't.

Most products work on the surface of the skin, that's true . . . but that doesn't mean they're not doing you any good. Products don't have to penetrate to the dermal layer to have an effect on the appearance of your skin. They can keep cells in the epidermis from drying out before they reach the surface; by plumping them, they can give the skin an added cushion, a little elasticity, fill in lines and elicit a very young, glowing look. These products really do this—they do make your skin look better! So they don't erase wrinkles . . . so what, if what they do do is improve (dramatically, used consistently!) the look of your skin.

What's more (and I think this is important in the way you think of caring for your skin), you should understand that though the top layer of your skin is dead in the strictest sense, it really isn't dead in the figurative sense. The way a skin-care expert explained it makes it very clear: Top-layer skin cells are dead in the same way a cut flower is dead; it's still a living thing—it has just been cut from its life support and (this is crucial), depending how it's cared for, it can thrive, even though it has lost its ability to regenerate.

And the fact of the matter is that many of the products don't just work on the surface layer of the skin; they penetrate and they do have the ability to speed cellular metabolism that has been slowed by time, stress, smoking and too much alcohol. Plus, improvements are being made all the time.

I can't tell you which product to buy because you are your own best skin-care expert . . . or you should be. Only you can really tell if a product is doing its job, because only you can see how your skin is reacting to the product twenty-four hours a day and know how it's working (better? worse?) in comparison to another product. (I believe in comparison shopping: No two skins are the same.) Of course the more you know about certain treatments and products, the better you'll know what to expect. Coming right up: all the basics on cleansing, toning, moisturizing, masks and exfoliating—how each works and what works best for what skin types in winter and in summer. Since Catherine has dry skin and I have oily (and we think we know what we're doing!), we'll divulge all our skin-care secrets.

Never, ever, no matter what you read, do facial exercises. Why? Because exercising facial muscles pulls facial skin, and pulling facial skin creates wrinkles (and if you doubt it, take a look at a stroke victim whose muscles are paralyzed on one side of the face only; that side can look ten to twenty years younger than the other). The same holds true for facial massage, though a gentle one to rev up circulation during a facial is fine—just make sure it's gentle!

BEFORE YOU BEGIN

I always check the label for ingredients I may be allergic to, and I think you should, too. Ingredients are listed in order of predominance, the greatest first. The ones most likely to cause irritation are the perfumes; if you're allergic to a fragrance, there are good unscented products to choose among.

After perusing the label, I screen new products on the inside of my elbow crease, an extremely sensitive (but inconspicuous) spot. I leave it on for twenty-four hours, and if it stings, burns or causes a rash, I don't use it.

But if I determine that I'm neither allergic nor sensitive to a product, I go ahead and test it. I always use a product for a couple weeks to see how it makes my skin look. (It usually takes a few weeks to see results.) Or sometimes I'll make simultaneous comparisons over several weeks, using one product on one side of my face, another on the other, before I use it regularly. (You can get sample sizes or buy travel sizes.) You might as well use the best possible product for your own skin.

CLEANSING

What It Can Do for You

One thing I notice is that the older a woman gets, the more likely she is to use more makeup and more moisturizer, making cleansing more important than ever.

A buildup of soot, dust, makeup, sweat and sebum makes for dull, lackluster skin (to say nothing of broken-out, irritated skin). When this "dirt" remains on the skin, proper cleansing is essential in helping skin regulate its water/oil balance, maintain its suppleness and help it to better absorb treatment products.

How to Cleanse

There are basically two schools of thought on the cleansing issue. One holds true to the old-fashioned soap-and-water-is-best theory; the other maintains that creamy cleansers are better. The first step in proper cleansing is determining which school you'll follow—or if you'll follow both. Actually, what

One of the best cleansers of all: a professional facial—one that includes a steaming to open pores, then a deep-pore cleansing and a peeling and/or moisturizing/conditioning mask. If you live in a polluted city, schedule one every month; if you don't, three to four times a year (or when seasons change) is ample. To note: Fingers are better than machines; gentle is always best— a good facial will leave your skin smooth and glowing, not red and irritated.

it boils down to is a matter of preference (what you feel works best for you), though, generally speaking, normal-to-oily skin may do better with soap and water and normal-to-dry skin may do better with creamy cleansers, which are usually more emollient, less drying than soap. Either way, don't overdo. Don't scrub too hard or use a too-harsh product or you'll dry skin, cause irritation, even breakouts.

About soap and water: soap is a very effective cleanser, usually leaving skin feeling squeaky clean. It works by first chemically combining with dirt so the combination (dirt and soap) can be rinsed off easily. Water alone won't remove dirt, as you know; neither will soap alone.

Some people think that the pH of a soap will affect your skin, that you should go for a soap with a pH of 5 to 7, which won't irritate skin's neutral pH; but Albert M. Kligman, M.D., professor of dermatology, University of Pennsylvania School of Medicine, said he's done extensive research that proves the pH of a soap doesn't affect your skin in any way; that whatever soap you use, your skin will return to its neutral pH level soon after washing. My only recommendation: Never use a deodorant soap or a scented bath soap on your face—both are drying. Go for either a synthetic cleansing bar, transparent soap (made with at least 10 percent glycerin, a humectant that attracts moisture and draws it into your skin) or a superfatted soap (to which extra oils and/or emollients have been added to help lock in moisture).

The best way to cleanse with soap and water: Wash hands • Wet the soap and stroke the bar across your face • Wet hands and, using your fingertips, work up a lather on face and neck (whenever you wash your face, wash your neck, too), avoiding the eye area • Rinse thoroughly with lukewarm water—never hot, which opens pores to let moisture escape, expands capillaries and, over time, can lead to redness, blotchiness and obviously visible veins—and gently pat dry with a soft terry towel.

Note: No amount of rinsing is too much rinsing, especially if you live in a hard-water area—Chicago; Dallas; Houston; Los Angeles; Philadelphia; Minneapolis or Washington, D.C., for example. The metal ions in hard water combine with soap and leave a residue that can dull skin and prevent treatment products from doing their job. If your tap water is hard, double or triple your rinse time and consider buying bottled water for rinsing your face (soapy residue not only makes skin drab-looking, it can be irritating, too). Soft water, on the other hand, is beautifying (Atlanta, New Orleans, New York City, Savannah and Seattle are soft-water areas).

About cleansers: Creamy cleansers are effective, too. They don't dry or irritate skin. In fact, they're quite emollient and you have to be careful not to choose one that's so heavy it leaves a greasy residue that'll clog pores and prevent the absorption of moisturizers.

The best way to use a cleanser: With clean hands, simply use your fingertips to smooth on all over face and neck, avoiding the eye area • Use cotton balls or absorbent cotton pads to wipe off; keep changing cotton pads and wiping off cleanser until the pad doesn't have a trace of dirt on it • Do not use tissue, which is made from wood and can irritate skin • You don't need to rinse unless you are using one of the washing creams, which work the same way cleansing creams do but are water soluble and can easily be rinsed off.

Cleansing in Winter

Normal/dry skin: Because her skin tends to be dry anyway, Catherine cuts cleansing down to once a day—"twice, tops!"—during the dry winter months; and she uses a superemollient cleanser, never soap, which "strips away what natural moisture my skin does have."

At night (after removing her makeup), Catherine washes with her cleanser and a natural sponge that helps stimulate circulation. "In the morning I 'cleanse' with tepid water only, no cleanser—how could my skin have gotten dirty during the night?—at least a half-hour before leaving my apartment so there's no dampness to cause chapping. Even if when I wake up my skin feels slightly oily, I still splash only tepid water on my face. I don't use a cleanser because I don't want to lose the film of oil that's my own natural moisturizer and protection against dehydration and the elements!''

Normal/oily skin: I'm addicted to soap, even in winter. It's one of the things that keeps me from having a lot of blackheads and whiteheads. I use a milder soap during the cold dry months than I do in summer. To save time I do most of my skin-care routine in the shower. In the winter I keep my shower briefer than in the summer, so the prolonged exposure to water doesn't dehydrate my skin. (When skin is over hydrated, it begins to dehydrate rapidly as excess moisture evaporates.) I use soap morning and night, and I just keep putting my face under the shower head over and over until every last trace of it is gone. Bonus: I find this is a great skin circulation booster, too.

If you live in or are traveling to a polluted city . . . Skin will become dry and dirty *in winter* and so needs extra cleansing with a gentle soap or cleanser; and *in summer* it'll become oily and dirty and so needs extra cleansing with a stronger soap or cleanser, followed by an astringent or freshener.

Tip: Always use a moisturizer to serve as a barrier between your skin and pollution, which causes aging (see p. 62).

Cleansing in Summer

High humidity (which is great for all skin types) and high temperatures can make you feel sweaty and sticky, and you'll probably feel like cleansing several times a day. One thing both Catherine and I do after a particularly oppressive day—those New York City days in July and August when you could fry an egg on the pavement: We treat our faces to an herbal facial sauna to open pores, draw out impurities. Here's how: In a large pot, boil about 2 quarts of water with 3 generous teaspoons of Swiss Kriss herb leaves. Let it simmer for 3 minutes. Then remove it from the heat, cover your head with a towel and hold it over the pot, about 8 to 12 inches from the water, for 5 minutes. Splash your face with cold water to rinse off wastes.

Normal/dry skin: At night, in summer, Catherine switches to a superfatted soap, and she uses her creamy cleanser in the morning when there's not a lot of dirt or sweat to remove.

Normal/oily skin: In addition to my morning shower cleansing, at night I use a stronger cleanser, am sure to rinse well (to get my skin really clean) and then finish with an alcohol-based toner (since my skin is at its oiliest in summer).

TONING

What It Can Do for You

There's a lot of confusion about what toning is and does. Most women think toners only tighten pores. They do make pores *look* smaller (you can't change pore size), but most significantly, toners remove oil and dirt. Consider toning part two of your cleansing routine.

In addition, toning restores skin's acid mantle; effects a rosy glow as it brings blood to the surface to nourish and moisturize cells; leaves skin feeling cool and refreshed.

How to Tone

After cleansing (you'll be surprised what a toner will take off after you've cleansed) and/or for a quick cleanup, say, mid-afternoon and/or for a pick-me-up (toners are very refreshing, leave skin tingling), simply saturate a cotton ball and wipe off dirt. Remember, you are removing dirt, not putting on toner.

There are two types of toners: fresheners/toners, which are mild (with little or no alcohol) and good for normal-to-dry skin, especially in winter; and astringents, which are strong (with high concentrations of alcohol) and are good for oily skin, particularly in summer.

Toning in Winter

A winter rule of thumb (especially for dry skin): Avoid any product that contains alcohol.

Toning in Summer

Dry skin does not need a toner in summer. Oily skin does. One of my favorites: one part lemon juice to ten parts water. It makes my skin feel fresh and clean.

MOISTURIZING

What It Can Do for You

I want to make one thing clear here: The surface moisture in your skin is composed of water from the sweat glands and oil from the sebaceous glands. When you think of moisturizing, remember that you are trying to supplement the amount of water in your skin, not the amount of oil.

However, it's important to remember that as you age, your oil glands produce less oil, which means that there's less of a natural oil barrier to protect against evaporation of water produced by the sweat glands (whose production also slows with age). That's why moisturizing becomes increasingly important with age (and also why oily skin, which creates more of a protective barrier against moisture loss than dry skin, shows fewer and later signs of aging).

While some moisturizers act as a barrier to prevent moisture loss, sealing in what natural moisture your skin has, others act as humectants, drawing moisture in from the environment and adding it to the top layers of your skin, temporarily plumping dry surface cells. Neither, alone, is enough.

But there is a whole new breed of supermoisturizers available now that do more: They penetrate beneath the epidermis to moisturize the cells below, and they increase cell turnover, improve skin texture and diminish fine lines—that is, they physiologically affect the skin. The problem is finding a product that does all of this.

Recently I spoke to a skin research scientist, and here's how he told me to test a moisturizer's deep-penetrating potential and effectiveness: Stop using it for two weeks. If you're using a physiologically active product, your skin will continue to look moist and healthy (just as if you were continuing use of the product) during those two weeks. The reason: It takes two weeks for the cells in the outer layer of the skin to turn over and be replaced by the new fresh, moisturized cells. If you're using a moisturizer that acts only as a barrier, you'll notice drier, scalier skin within twenty-four hours after you stop using the product.

How to Moisturize

Once you find a deep-penetrating moisturizer that works for you, get into the habit of using it every morning after cleansing and toning, while your skin is still damp (so you seal in moisture) and before you put on the rest of your makeup; and every evening, too, after cleansing and toning, again while skin is still damp and at least twenty minutes before you go to bed to give it time to be absorbed by the skin so it won't rub off on your pillow.

Whatever you do, don't be fooled by the myth that your skin needs to breathe at night and so shouldn't be moisturized. It's difficult to make skin hold its breath.

On the other side of the coin, don't be taken in by the idea that the more moisturizer you slather on, the more you're lubricating your skin; you may end up just clogging your pores. How much is too much? Take a dime-size amount of cream and smooth it on your face and neck; if you run out before you finish, you're applying it too heavy-handedly.

Another common mistake: Many women think that the heavier the moisturizer they use, the more they're moisturizing their skin. Wrong! The dull, sallow appearance of some women's skin is due to their using a too-heavy moisturizer. The reason: The thicker the moisturizer (and the more of it you use), the slower the rate of cell turnover; when you use a too-heavy cream, you are actually slowing cell renewal because the reproductive cells in the basal layer "think" that the moisturizer is really a dead-skin layer and, to compensate, they produce fewer new cells to move up to replace them.

How to tell if you're using too rich a moisturizer: After you apply it, note how long it takes before your skin feels oily. If you apply it first thing in the morning and your forehead and cheeks feel greasy an hour or so later, that's a sure sign that you're using too rich a formulation. This can also happen with a foundation; switch to a formulation with less oil in it or look for a water-base foundation for oily or combination skin.

So what exactly should you use? A deep-penetrating moisturizer, to be sure. And, generally speaking, if you have dry skin you'll do better with a cream formulation; if you have oily skin you'll do better with lighter lotion formulations.

> Some experts feel that *extreme* dryness is caused by a low-grade inflammation of the skin. The new over-the-counter hydrocortisone creams are great for this problem. They penetrate, hydrate cells and reduce inflammation caused by dryness. Check with your dermatologist.

If you look at the ingredients in your moisturizer, you'll find that water is the first or second listed (remember that ingredients are listed in order of their predominance, greatest first). This might seem odd, since you don't want to spend money on water (though I have to say that one of the best ways to swell the outer layer of skin and temporarily smooth out wrinkles is to splash plain old water on your face). But water alone can't moisturize your skin; you need other ingredients. The water in the product is there to be absorbed by the skin; the oil is there to keep it from evaporating.

Moisturizing in Winter

Cold temperature and low humidity almost literally lift the moisture out of your skin, making it look more wrinkled than it really is (remember, moisture puffs up skin). Combine this with the fact that indoor heating can create an environment with a humidity level as low as that of the Sahara Desert, and you'll understand why I say so strongly: Dry or oily (but especially dry!), your skin needs a good moisturizer in winter—a heavier one used more frequently than the moisturizer you use in hot humid weather (it should be heavy enough to alleviate the dry, cracked, scaly feeling immediately).

Here are some special cold-weather moisturizing tips for dry skin from Catherine: She keeps a moisturizer in her desk during the dry winter months for a midday moisturizing. And on weeknights she moisturizes twice, once with her morning moisturizer as soon as she gets home, then again with a special night cream (see p. 67) about a half-hour before she goes to bed.

If your skin looks particularly dry and lined, here's a quick wrinkle remover: Massage a rich cream into your skin before showering or bathing.

Continue after you get into the shower or bath, working the cream into the skin on your face and neck until it's absorbed. Together, the moisturizer, the massage and the steam will puff up your lines.

Reminder: Don't overreact to winter dryness by overmoisturizing.

> Pregnant women, especially those in their thirties and forties, will find that their skin will change. The good news is that it will get a wonderful warm natural glow due to an increase in estrogen, which causes the blood vessels near the epidermis to dilate. The bad news: Skin will probably get abnormally dry because the sebaceous glands slow down, produce less sebum. The moral: Moisturize more!

Another moisturizing strategy Catherine takes in winter (and so do I as a preventive measure for my oily skin): a humidifier. It can make a major difference in how dry your skin gets. We prefer the inexpensive cold water vaporizers. Not only do they cost less, they're easily portable, easily cleanable and, because they're small and don't "store" water, bacteria never have a really good chance to develop in them and cause respiratory problems.

Both of us keep humidifiers going in our apartments all the time during the winter, and at work most editors keep a pan of water on the radiator or use a small humidifier. You should also use plants as natural humidifiers in your office or at home: Ferns are the best choice—fill a tray with pebbles, set potted plants on top and add water to the top of the pebbles.

Note: The relative humidity of skin is 87 percent. Heated rooms in winter and air-conditioned rooms in summer have humidities as low as 30 percent—one good reason to use a humidifier in summer as well as winter.

Moisturizing in Summer

Even though all skin types may feel hydrated in hot weather (high temperatures melt the oily film on the skin's surface, which, when combined with perspiration, makes skin feel moist), everyone—even the oiliest skin types—should still moisturize. *Special tips for oily skin:* I make sure I choose the lightest product I can find, because I know anything else will just sit on the surface of my skin, make it shiny and highlight my lines! I find lotions are generally better than creams on my oily skin in summer. As you probably know, besides turning hot air cold, air-conditioners make hot, muggy air habitable by lowering its humidity—the result, obviously, being drier skin. And if I find shine, I degleam my face with a special paper blotter I keep handy in my purse and desk drawer.

A word of caution to swimmers: Chlorinated pool water robs skin of its surface oil protection. To protect all skin types, apply a moisturizer before swimming. After swimming, cleanse with a gentle soap or cleanser and follow with a light moisturizer.

More on Moisturizing

EYE CREAMS

I'm often asked why you need a special cream for your eyes. There are a few very good reasons: The skin around the eyes is extremely thin, contains no oil glands, is more sensitive to certain ingredients (fragrances, for example) than is the skin on the rest of the face and it is, therefore, subject to the first signs of aging. Eye creams are specially formulated for this delicate area with penetrating oils that will keep the skin around the eyes well lubricated and soft but without being so oily that they seep into your eyes. They also create a fine film, which deflects light and actually diminishes the appearance of fine lines.

Tip: Make sure the cream you choose doesn't leave too heavy a film because (1) you'll want to be able to apply makeup over it, and (2) you don't want any shine that'll enhance your lines.

Use eye creams gently! Pat—never pull—with the pad of your middle or index fingertip in two or three small circles at the outer corner of the eyes (where lines usually show up first . . . and become deepest) and work toward the inner corner of the eye, up the inside of the nose, over the lid and brow area and back to the outer corner.

Eye creams should be used in winter and summer, on dry and oily skin types . . . everyone should use eye creams every day, morning and night.

THROAT CREAMS

Like eye creams, these are specially formulated: Because the skin on the neck has fewer oil glands than the skin on the face, I think it's a good idea to use a heavier cream here—you need to keep it well lubricated to keep lines at

> **Do the New Antiwrinkle Products Work?**
> A whole new product category has emerged, making strong promises of being able to repair—youthen, if you will—old-looking skin. Do they work?
>   Antiwrinkle products will not remove what lines you have. But here's what they will do: They will make the lines you have look less conspicuous by plumping and firming the skin around them, improving the skin's microcirculation. And—this is important!—they can actually keep the lines you will get from being as "bad" as they might be if you weren't using the product. The reason: These new products will help speed the skin's natural cell renewal-repair process.

bay. As I've said before, the neck is an oft-neglected area and one that does need special care. A special throat cream should be added to your moisturizing regimen if for no other reason than it'll make you remember your neck!

Tip: Always apply upward from your collarbone to your chin.

HORMONE CREAMS

With small amounts of hormones like estrogen in them, these creams promise to help postmenopausal women with excessively dry skin. But according to Darrell Rigel, M.D., a New York City dermatologist, hormone creams can't do any more than a regular moisturizer. The hormone molecule cannot pass through the skin. My feeling is: Why fool around with them when there are so many effective creams on the market.

NIGHT CREAMS

I'm sure you know that while you're sleeping, some bodily functions slow—the heart rate, blood pressure and breathing rate, for example. But did you also know that the body is extra busy manufacturing hormones, enzymes and other body chemicals needed to replace those that are lost or used up during the day? And that the skin's cell regeneration rate peaks and its metabolism functions at its highest level during the night? (If you doubt it, take a look at your skin after a few sleepless nights; I'm sure you'll notice it looks less healthy and glowing.)

Night creams are in part responsible for how effectively skin cells reproduce, because they stimulate the skin's own regenerative process to function more effectively. Plus, they bind moisture within the skin so that when you awaken, your skin looks softer and fine surface lines are minimized.

FIRMING CREAMS

As I said in the beginning of this chapter, no product is going to unwrinkle wrinkled skin, but these creams contain ingredients that will improve the appearance of old-looking skin by improving microcirculation and toning and tightening the epidermis.

OXYGENATING PRODUCTS

Though your skin gets most of its oxygen (necessary for healthy, young-looking skin) from the bloodstream, it does absorb about $2^1/_2$ percent of the body's total oxygen from the air . . . and it eliminates about 3 percent of the body's carbon dioxide waste, too. You've probably heard exercise experts talk about breathing correctly to extend your endurance capability; think of it this way, too: Every time you inhale and exhale, you're breathing for younger-looking skin! But, as you get older, your skin's ability to take in oxygen from the air weakens. What happens to skin cells that don't get enough oxygen: The epidermis begins to thin; your skin looks drier, duller; there's a slowing of the cell turnover rate, loss of elasticity . . . and more rapid aging of the cells.

Now available over the counter are special oxygenating products that stimulate the skin's oxygen-absorption capabilities. Don't worry about using them when you're too young: You can't oversupply your cells with oxygen; what they don't need, they don't take in. Two more easy ways to get oxygen to

---

Do Ampoules Work?

In my opinion, yes.

Tiny vials of concentrated ingredients that may moisturize, nourish or rejuvenate, ampoules are a kind of shock treatment for the skin because they aren't used daily and your skin is not accustomed to them.

Catherine uses moisturizing ampoules on her dry skin every three months or so, and I use cell rejuvenation ampoules between seasons to stimulate cell renewal.

the skin cells: doing a headstand for two minutes daily or taking a brisk half-hour walk.

MASKS

What They Can Do for You

I feel toning-tightening and moisturizing masks are an absolute must. (There are also peeling—exfoliating—masks, which I'll get to on p. 54).

Moisturizing masks hydrate the skin in one of two ways—either they create an impenetrable barrier that forces water into the cells or they supplement moisture through osmosis.

Toning-tightening masks are smoothed on and, as they harden, they constrict the skin. When they're rinsed or peeled off, pores look smaller (because the constricted blood vessels then expand, giving skin a pink, plumped-up appearance without lines).

The effects of these masks are not necessarily long-lasting, but as a temporary lift, masks will not only give you a physical boost but a psychological one, too.

How to Use Masks

Think of masks as weekly or bi-weekly supplements to your regular toning and moisturizing routines. Try to set aside ten minutes or so when you're relaxed. Apply the mask to thoroughly cleaned, still-damp skin; or, better yet, steam your face to open pores before applying. Always avoid the eye area (I use an eye cream for protection). While the mask is on, lie down and place cotton pads soaked with witch hazel or rosewater over your eyes. To remove: Soak cotton in cool water and use a gentle upward motion. Finish with a moisturizer, even if you've just used a moisturizing mask.

Tip: When you're pressed for time, try using a mask while you're showering—it's a great skin booster.

Masks for All Seasons

Whatever type of mask you use, be aware that what's important are its ingredients, not its form (e.g., gel or cream). Here are some guidelines (not hard-and-fast rules).

If you have normal/dry skin: Go for mineral or vegetable oils, placenta, aloe vera, panthenol, carotene and collagen. Avoid oil-absorbing ingredients such as kaolin, talc and oatmeal.

If you have normal/oily skin: Go for clay, aloe vera, ginseng, yeast and calamine. Avoid oils and fragrances.

Note: If you're acne prone, steer clear of masks that contain grains, which are abrasive and inhibit healing.

If your skin is sensitive (whether dry or oily): Go for rose hips, panthenol, allantoin and chamomile. Avoid silicates, alcohol, kelp and sulfur.

Here are some year-round mask recipes both Catherine and I love to whip up ourselves.

Mask Recipes for All Seasons

TONING

THE EGG-WHITE MASK

After a long day at work, before an evening out, I apply this tightening mask.

1 egg white

Whip in a bowl. Apply to skin. Let dry and rinse with tepid water.

THE BASIC BUTTERMILK PICK-ME-UP MASK

When my skin looks pasty and pale mid-winter, this mask from Ole Henriksen, a Los Angeles skin-care expert, always comes to my rescue. It seems to plump up my skin, erase my lines, too.

¼-½ cup thick buttermilk

Simply massage buttermilk over face and neck. Leave on for 20 to 30 minutes; rinse with tepid water. Moisturize.

MOISTURIZING

THE EGG-AND-HONEY MASK

When Catherine's skin is particularly dry and chapped, she uses this mask twice a week.

1 egg yolk
2 tablespoons honey

Whisk ingredients together until a smooth paste forms. Smooth onto the face and neck. Leave on for 20 minutes; rinse with tepid water. Moisturize.

THE THREE-OIL SKIN SMOOTHER

This mask from New York City skin-care expert Lia Schorr works best after exfoliating. When the dead cells are gone, the oils will penetrate deeper and effect smoother, softer, more glowing skin.

¼ cup olive oil   ¼ cup sesame oil
¼ cup almond oil   Absorbent cotton

Combine the oils in a small saucepan and whisk together over low heat. Remove from stove when warm.

Take a sheet of absorbent cotton big enough to fit over your face and neck and soak it in the oil; squeeze out excess and apply to the skin. Leave on for 20 minutes. Cleanse and rinse with lukewarm water.

YOGURT MASK

Easy as can be—and, as if that weren't enough, it's super soothing to sunburn pain and helps guard against broken capillaries that are often more severe in summer's heat than in winter, too.

½ cup plain yogurt

Simply slather on face, leave on for 15 minutes and rinse off with cold water.

EXFOLIATION

What It Can Do for You

Since I started exfoliating four years ago, I've seen a major change in my skin: I no longer have blackheads, my skin is smoother and it looks healthier than it's ever looked.

Exfoliating can give you a new skin in a matter of minutes! Sloughing off dead, dull surface cells exposes a new, younger-looking, smooth and even layer of skin cells that absorb and reflect light, so lines look softer and skin glows. (If light hits a smooth surface it bounces off as a perfect, even reflection; if it hits a rough surface it creates shadows and the surface looks duller and older.)

Exfoliation also can actually speed the cell renewal rate by 30 percent. Here's why: Every twenty-five to thirty days your skin renews itself—it sloughs off its outermost layer of about a million dull, dried-out dead cells (among the 100 million cells on your face) and replaces it with a brand new layer of healthy moisture-plump cells that have been generated deep in the dermis. This natural sloughing process slows naturally as you get older and, in addition, it's stymied by the ravages of the environment—sun, wind, pollution, dirt and makeup, all of which combine to age the topmost layer of cells faster than new cells can be produced to replace them. Thus, old-looking surface cells linger longer than they should and give your skin a dull, lifeless appearance, to say nothing of interfering with the generation of new cells. That's where exfoliation comes in (and it explains, too, why men's skin is often so much better-looking at the same age as women's—their daily shaving is daily exfoliating).

How to Exfoliate

There are several methods of exfoliation. Which you choose is a matter of personal preference, but all should be done gently so as not to irritate or damage skin.

Tip: One way to make sure that you're not applying too much pressure is to keep your thumbs under your chin and use the other four fingers to exfoliate.

1. *The chemical method.* An exfoliant (usually containing salicylic acid) is spread on the skin and dissolves the dead surface cells as well as skin oils that otherwise glue together surface cells. These exfoliants are usually best for normal/oily skin types.

2. *The mechanical method.* A scrub derived from natural (ground apricot pits, almonds or oatmeal) or synthetic ingredients is massaged onto the face to loosen and then lift dead cells. The scrub can either be a mask you put on, let dry and then rub off; or a cream you put on wet skin and rub for one minute. Tip: Look for products with relatively uniform small grains, which work gently, easily. Or try simply rubbing papaya pulp or pineapple slices on your face—they're both extremely gentle, natural exfoliants.

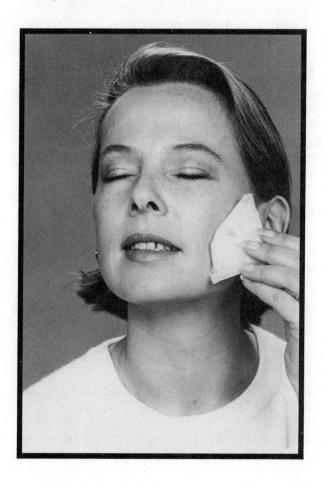

3. Another mechanical method involves synthetic exfoliating *sponges* you use with soap and water or cleanser to whisk away the top layer of the skin.

When to Exfoliate

Regardless of your skin type, you should exfoliate every day (if not twice a day). But if you haven't been exfoliating, you have to build up to a regular daily routine slowly (it may take about a month)—say 15 seconds in the morning and 15 seconds at night, gradually increasing to 30 seconds each time until you reach one minute.

Tip: If your skin starts to look red and feel sensitive, you're doing too much and need to cut back. Try just a few seconds every day until your skin feels comfortable, and then begin to increase the time.

Exfoliating in Winter

Normal/dry skin: Not all flaking is chapping! Skin, especially dry skin, is in a constant state of irritation due to cold, dry air, and it compensates by turning over cells at a relatively rapid rate. That's why even Catherine, with her dry skin, exfoliates every day in winter. She uses a sea sponge with a gentle cream-based scrub to remove dead skin cells without taking the skin's protective mantle with it.

Normal/oily skin: With my oily skin, I've gotten into the habit of exfoliating at least once, often twice a day during winter. Here's what I do: Since exfoliation is most effective on thoroughly cleansed skin (so it concentrates not on the surface grime but on the cells underneath), I find it best to exfoliate in the shower, where I can pre-steam my face and soften surface cells so they're easier to lift off; then I tone and finish with a light moisturizer. What I've found is that flaking stops and my skin looks softer, much better hydrated.

Exfoliating in Summer

Because skin thickens with sun exposure—and, in fact, often peels—daily exfoliation is an absolute necessity (not a luxury) for *both dry and oily skin types,* especially at the very end of summer when you cut down on your time outdoors and the cell turnover rate that might otherwise push away dead, dull top-layer cells slows with melanin production. Many times after you've been in the sun all summer and your tan fades, you're left with an uneven skin tone . . . and you should consider having a mild chemical peel. Or ask your dermatologist about Retin-A, which acts as an exfoliator while it increases cell turnover (see p. 216).

Travel tip: Once I forgot my exfoliator on a week-long trip to the Caribbean. My skin was looking dull and drab. Here's how I improvised (and it really worked well): I saved one pack of sugar from my morning coffee, mixed it with my moisturizer until a granular paste formed, and rubbed it on my face as I would my regular exfoliating product. Then I simply washed, then rinsed and looked better than new!

A professional deep-pore cleansing will also help loosen and remove dead surface skin cells. Catherine has a standing appointment with her aesthetician the day after Labor Day for a special postsummer peeling mask. And I go to my aesthetician every three weeks for two or three months after Labor Day.

Note: Avoid exfoliating if your skin is sunburned, irritated or broken out, or if you've had a facial in the last day or two.

SPECIAL WINTER SKIN-CARE PRECAUTIONS

- *Consider the windchill factor,* which can be significantly lower than the actual temperature and means exposed skin can freeze more rapidly than expected. (Frostbite can be extremely damaging!) If, say, the temperature is 10° F and the wind speed is 15 mph, then the wind chill temperature is −18° F and likely to freeze exposed skin.
- *Double up on skin care and protection* if you're going to be outdoors in the extreme cold (and/or wind). What this means: two layers of moisturizer, two layers of sun screen, two coats of eye cream . . . all applied at least a half-hour (preferably at least an hour) before you go out.
- *Follow the Tan Plan in Chapter 7* if you're skiing (or doing anything outdoors, for that matter).
- *Note Catherine's skin-saving tips for skiers* (and use them, too, whenever you're going to be outdoors for any extended period of time): (1)

Want a good facial? Looking for a qualified aesthetician? Contact Aestheti-cians International, a nationwide association of dedicated professionals who are leaders in the field of skin-care services:

Mary Ann Graffeo, president
Aestheticians International Association
28 South Evergreen
Arlington Heights, IL 60005
(312) 259-9019

Reapply sun screen (SPF 15 or higher) frequently, especially if you're falling a lot and/or perspiring. (This, of course, after applying your initial two layers at least a half-hour before going outside.) (2) Ditto for special eye and lip sun screens. (3) Wear goggles or dark polarized sunglasses with eye guards that keep out sun and wind. (4) Wear baseball-cap hats—woolen ones over earmuffs in winter, canvas ones in spring. Their brims shield sun better than traditional ski hats. Tip: If you buy the hat in a children's store, the brim will be short enough so the wind won't catch under it and blow it off. (5) When it's snowing, cover your face by pulling your hat down on your forehead, wearing goggles and a neck gaiter pulled up over your mouth and nose (or wear a face mask whenever it's snowing or really cold). Skiing fast into snow breaks down the protective barrier on your skin, and the velocity whips away moisture, too. (6) Stay away from lodge fires—intense heat following exposure to cold air and wind can break capillaries. (7) Resist the urge to take a sauna after skiing—it will just be doubly drying in an already cold, dry environment. If you find you can't, do yourself this favor: Do not go into the sauna with a moisturizing cream on your face or body. Contrary to what you may have heard, it will not be easily absorbed; instead it will clog pores and inhibit perspiration. The time to moisturize is when your sauna is over.

Prevent lips from chapping with constant coverage with an opaque lipstick, a product like zinc oxide or a lip balm with an SPF of at least 10. Just get in the habit of applying protection immediately after your morning shower and again and again throughout the day. FYI: The reason lips are so prone to chapping in winter is that the dry air tends to make you lick them; the more you do, the drier they become as the moisture evaporates.

- *Don't forget eyes!* It goes almost without saying that the delicate skin around eyes, so susceptible to dryness, needs extra care in winter. What works to keep the eye area well lubricated: in the A.M., a gel, a sheer emollient stick or a very light cream that doesn't smudge makeup, blur vision or sting eyes; midday, a reapplication if you've been outside for a half-hour or more, or if it's particularly cold and windy; in the P.M., a richer, thicker cream than you used in the morning.

    Tip: Apply in a sweeping motion away from the edge of lids, where capillary action might pull the lubricant into the eye, possibly causing irritation.

SPECIAL SUMMER SKIN-CARE PRECAUTIONS

- *Rinse away potentially drying chlorine.* Keep a spray bottle of mineral water in your bag; be sure to dry skin completely after spraying or your face may chap.
- *Don't spritz off saltwater.* In spite of all you've heard about saltwater drying out skin and hair, now it's thought that many of its minerals (iodine in particular) actually boost skin cells' oxygen intake and so up cell renewal. The result: healthier-looking, younger-looking, more glowing skin. Bonus: Sea air does the same trick (so even if you're not hot on swimming, you can still reap seawater's benefits).
- *Follow our Tan Plan religiously!* (see Chapter 7.)

THE ANTIWRINKLE TRAVELER'S GUIDE

Many women notice a change in their skin when they travel, but they don't do anything about it. They just chalk up their too-dry or too-oily skin to the food or the water and assume it'll return to normal when they get home—a big mistake, because over time (especially if you travel frequently), skin that's "too anything" will look less than its best.

The reason your skin changes when you travel is that the climate has changed, and just as you adjust your skin-care routine to seasonal changes, so you should adjust it to different climates. And this is particularly true the older you get: As you age, skin doesn't adapt as readily to climatic changes as it did when you were young.

What happens to skin when you go from cold to hot: Most noticeably, it is better hydrated than in cold weather, because the air itself is more humid and, additionally, heat stimulates oil glands, which produce a protective (and lubricating) film on the surface of the skin and so make skin stronger, thicker, too • Because your skin has not been acclimated to the sun, it is more susceptible to burning.

What happens to skin when you go from hot to cold: • Cold air constricts blood vessels, slowing circulation and decreasing the amount of oxygen and nutrients the skin cells receive • Low humidity and high wind increase evaporation of skin's moisture, thereby causing dehydration • Sebaceous glands are less active in cold weather than in hot, contributing further to the dehydration problem and making skin thinner, more vulnerable to the elements, too (because there is no adequate protective oil barrier between the skin and the elements).

To the rescue: the winter tips throughout this chapter if you're heading to a cold climate; the summer tips if you're going south.

And while you're on the way, here are a few beautifiers for fliers that really work!

- Before you go, wash your face and apply a rich moisturizer (if you have very dry skin, apply your night cream) while skin is still damp—it'll serve as a barrier against the dirty dry-air supply in the cabin.
- Carry a spray can of water and spray yourself every half-hour or so, and drink at least four 8-ounce glasses of water during a five-hour trip.
- Wear rich eye cream, which can double as a lip balm to keep lips moist, too. Reapply every hour (after your spritzing).
- Don't wear makeup (apply it right before you're going to land instead)—it'll just make your skin feel dirty and, if you are lucky enough to be able to fall asleep, eye makeup will just get into your eyes and you'll wind up looking awful.
- Refrain from alcohol, coffee, too—both will cause puffiness, dehydrate your skin.

FOUR

MAKING UP

(FOR LOST TIME)

There's something about aging that changes the way women think about makeup. They almost always react in one of two ways: Either they feel that makeup accentuates their lines and they opt to wear no makeup at all, or they go to the other extreme and, in an attempt to cover their lines, they apply too much makeup. Both approaches are all wrong. My personal taste is something in the middle of these extremes—a natural look that enhances what's strong, hides what's wrong.

> With the right amount of makeup in the right colors applied with the right techniques, you can camouflage lines and hold off plastic surgery for at least ten years.

The next 36 pages are devoted to showing you how correct, well-blended makeup tones will soften every line, drawing attention away from wrinkles. Eyes and brows, cheeks and face and lips are each treated separately, with their own easy-to-follow application techniques and color suggestions.

But before beginning, I want to stress the importance of investing in the right makeup tools. No matter what product you use, no matter how well you've mastered the application concepts, if you don't have the right tools, your makeup will be messy and too heavy (brushes give a lighter application than fingers)—and nothing is more aging than sloppy, heavy-handed makeup.

Here's everything you'll need for young-looking makeup—the best anti-aging investment you can make.

- eye shadow brush
- eyeliner brush
- lip brush
- brow brush (with eyelash comb)

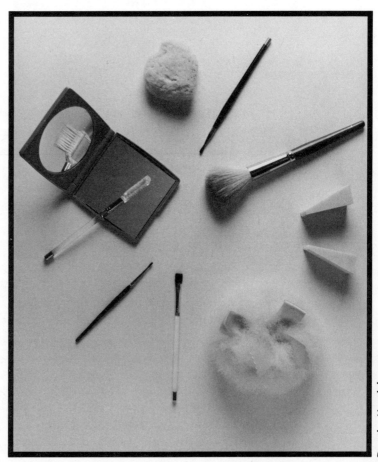

Dorothy Handelman

- blusher brush
- powder brush
- powder puff
- a few small sponges (including a silk sponge—naturally porous with the texture of silk—to apply foundation; a circle sponge—dense rubber with a smooth surface—to apply blusher; a diamond sponge—dense rubber with straight wedge—to smooth makeup under eyes and around nose)
- makeup mirror with magnifying side

THE RIGHT LIGHT FOR MAKING UP . . . AND AFTER

Applying makeup in the wrong light is one of the primary reasons for too-heavily-applied colors.

So that you can see what you're doing and correct any mistakes (too much blusher is the most common one), here are the makings of the most effective makeup light.

- Ideally, light should come from three sources—overhead and from both sides of the mirror.
- It should be directed at the face, not reflected outward from the mirror, which will produce glare, or upward from the sink or counter, which will deceptively fill in unattractive shadows.
- Use incandescent or soft-white fluorescent lamps, which will enhance reds, yellows and oranges and "warm" the face. A lot of celebrities use pink bulbs for a warm, flattering glow! Stay away from cool-white fluorescent lamps, which have a graying effect.
- Dimmers are great—they can simulate the light you'll be in (high noon or a candlelit dinner) and let you check your makeup for absolute accuracy.

It should go without saying that no matter how carefully you make yourself up, if you don't consider the light you'll be seen in, all the effort will have been in vain. Here are some general guidelines to keep in mind.

If you're going to be in daylight, plan ahead: Makeup may look heavy, so use a light hand. Gels and creams are your best bet (powders can make your skin look dry). Go for pink lips and cheeks, beige and brown shades for the eyes; stay away from pasty pastels and too-bold brights.

If you're going to be indoors, in, say, an office, you could get into trouble! There are no red rays in fluorescent light, making colors with a blue base (like fuchsia, magenta, burgundy) your best bet. Avoid yellow and red and any makeup with built-in sheen. Consider, too, that because fluorescent light makes darks look darker, your blush should be lighter, as should your lipstick and lip liner.

If you're going to be in low light, in the evening, for example, think pale and pink (especially if you're going to be in candlelight). Colors appear darker in low light, the reason dramatic evening makeup often looks cheap.

QUICK COSMETIC EYE-LIFTS

Because the skin around the eyes is thin and lacks oil glands, it tends to wrinkle before the rest of the face. Crow's-feet, droopy and sagging lids and undereye lines are common—but they can be camouflaged with the right makeup. Here's how.

To Eliminate Fine Lines and Crow's-Feet

- Simply use an undereye concealer or foundation close to your own skin tone. Stay away from white, which will enhance, not hide, lines.
- Stick to matte eye shadows in soft muted colors like taupe, brown, gray and mauve. Frosted shadows will always accentuate lines.
- Use cream shadows if you're very lined: They cover lines, while powder shadows get caught in them.
- Don't apply your eye shadow beyond the eye, where it will highlight crow's-feet and undereye lines.
- Line your eyes with soft brown liner and smudge it. Stay away from black, which is aging.

> Keep this artistic rule of thumb in mind: Dark colors make lines recede; light ones make them more prominent.

To Camouflage Crepey, Droopy Lids

- So that you never have creased, caked or faded shadow, always use an eye shadow base.
- To visually uplift droopy lids, layer your shadow: Apply a thin layer of medium brown matte shadow from lashes to brows; then, on the lid, a softer, lighter taupe or mauve shadow. Both these brown-based colors tend to make the crepey part of the lid recede.
- Concentrate your eye shadow on the outer half of your lids to give a wide-eyed, youthful appearance (below, left).
- For the most natural look, apply a dark foundation on the lids instead of eyeshadow.
- If your lids are excessively crepey, go for liner instead of cream shadows—it's less likely to seep into creases. Line the entire eye (upper and lower lids near the lash line) with a dark brown liner and smudge it with a soft eye shadow brush.
- Open sagging eyes instantly: Curl lashes and apply two coats of mascara on upper lashes, one on lower lashes. (Heavy mascara on lower lashes creates an aging shadow.)
- To give definition to droopy lids, line with a very dark brown liner under upper lashes (below, right).
- You can also have eyelashes dyed. Pluses: This is great in summer, when you may not want to wear mascara, say, at the beach; avoids eye wear and tear (especially from not having to remove mascara). Minuses: lasts only three weeks; isn't as eye defining as two coats of mascara because it only colors, doesn't thicken.

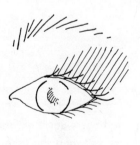 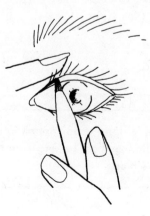

Margaret A. Hinders

Instead of lining eyes—on crepey lids eyeliner can look uneven (and unsightly)—consider one of the new lash definer procedures now being done by many doctors across the country. Here's how it works (see opposite for the results): By injecting pigment into the dermis of the eyelid, the doctor tattoos tiny dots between the lashes, taking into consideration each client's coloring (on a woman with fair skin, he'd make light dots with a light gray or brown, while on a black or Oriental woman, he'd make heavier dots in dark brown or black). Done under local anesthesia, the procedure takes 30 minutes for upper lids, 45 for upper and lower; studies indicate that it lasts a lifetime. Here you can see how natural and eye-defining this procedure is. These young-looking eyes were done by Frank S. Socha, M.D., a New York City ophthalmologist and eye surgeon.

To Hide Bags and Undereye Circles

- Apply creamy undereye concealer. Try pale blue concealers, which cast shadows away from the face. Use a light touch, or it'll get caught in the creases. Be sure it's light textured, too.
- Another option: Just use a foundation that's a shade darker than the one you use on your face.
- Whatever you use, apply to the darkest part of the bag or circle and never right under lower lashes. (See right.)

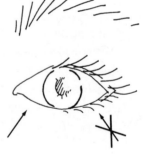

Margaret A. Hinders

Eyelining tip: a good controllable way to put on liner—dot it on, then blend the dots together, making sure there's no space between the lash line and the eyeliner.

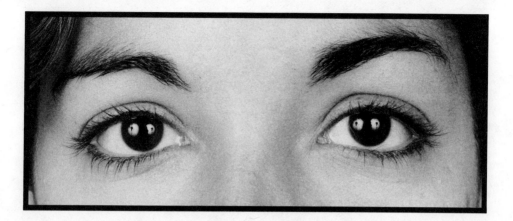

Colored Contacts Can Take Ten Years Off Your Looks

As you age, a yellow-white or gray ring forms around the colored part of your eye, the iris, making your eye look dull, older-looking. In effect, this ring, called the corneal arcus, is what's responsible for your losing your youthful twinkle. It's frequently inherited, but by the age of sixty, almost everyone has this condition.

. . . And everyone can minimize its appearance with tinted soft contact lenses (hard lenses are too small to cover the corneal arcus). On dark eyes, when the arcus—and aging—are most visible, amber or green lenses restore a youthful sparkle; on light eyes, any color—green, blue, aqua or amber—will match the arcus.

Here are three companies that make colored contact lenses:

· CTL Laboratories
· Bausch & Lomb
· Ciba Vision Care

To Brighten Tired Eyes

• Soft pastel shadows will give you a fresher look when you're tired than dark, dramatic colors.

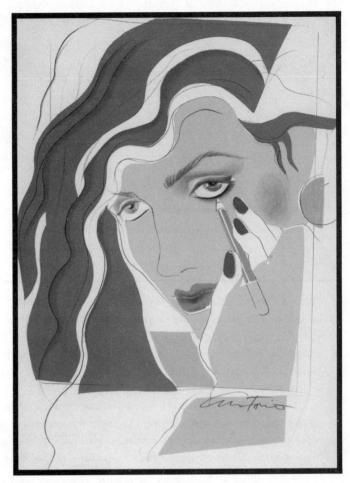

Don't underline
the whole eye

- If you use liner under bottom lashes, be sure to use it just three-quarters of the way across the eye, from the outer corner in, not all the way to the nose. If you line from corner to corner, you'll create a too-heavy look.

   Tip: Don't draw the line too close to the iris or you'll make the eye look small; droopy, too.
- Consider blue liner—it'll draw redness out of the white of the eyes, actually make whites appear cleaner, brighter.
- Blue mascara just on the tips of upper lashes brightens eyes. You should apply it right over black or brown mascara.

• After you've finished applying your blusher, brush whatever is left on the brush under the browbone—you'll be surprised how it'll "light up" your eyes.

UPLIFTING BROWS

Many women neglect their brows . . . but don't you! Eyebrows are a distinctive feature (just think of the women whose brows helped make their faces famous—Audrey Hepburn, Brooke Shields, Mariel and Margaux Hemingway, to name a few).

Properly shaped brows can not only make a beautiful frame for eyes, they can also call attention away from wrinkles. On the other hand, an untweezed brow can compound the visual effects of droopy lids or lined eyes, and thin brows are always aging, since brow hair commonly thins through the years. Then, too, there's the myth of the brow that "lifts" the eye at the outer corner. Wrong. Those brows drawn with a pencil only draw attention to wrinkles because they're so fake-looking. Anything artificial will attract attention to details you want to hide. Follow these four simple steps and you'll be surprised at how much your brows can do for you.

1. Shape brows. The arch should peak slightly outside the pupil of the eye. Pluck hairs underneath so the brows are raised. The entire brow should end just at the outside corner of the eye and begin just above each side of the nose. And remember, too thin or too thick is immediately aging.
2. Give eyes an instant lift by brushing the brows up (not out). You can use a bit of eyebrow glue or petroleum jelly to keep them in place. Or put a small amount of hair gel on a brow brush and brush brows into place. (See next page.)
3. Your eyebrows should be one shade lighter than your hair color. (Gray is an exception; brows should be one shade darker than gray hair.) If your eyebrows are too dark, lighten them with a facial-hair bleach at home, or go to a salon. Too light? Darken your brows with a taupe or light brown brow pencil. Steer clear of dark brown or black pencils, which are too harsh.

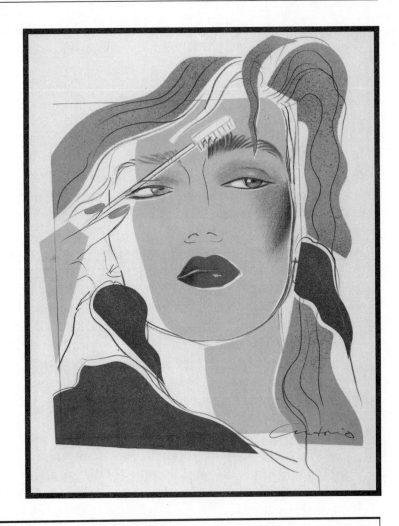

News! For women who have sparse brow hairs, say, from chronic plucking, almost no brow hair (common with age), or who have downward-sloping brows: A new eyebrow implant has been developed by Ian S. Brown, M.D., a Beverly Hills plastic surgeon. Under a local anesthetic, he actually tattoos eyebrows directly onto the skin with dyes specially mixed to match the patient's hair color.

He also uses this procedure to redefine lips so lipstick won't bleed into vertical lines and to repigment lost color on lips.

EYE-LIFTING EYEGLASSES

As soon as they start wearing glasses, some women stop wearing makeup because they think their eyes are no longer clearly visible; other women just continue wearing the same makeup they wore before. Both reactions are big mistakes.

Eyes can be seen through glasses, so don't go bare-eyed—it's as important to cover wrinkles if you wear glasses as it is if you don't. And once you don glasses, you ought to consider changing your makeup. Here's why:

If *you're nearsighted*, your lenses are thin at the edges, thick in the middle. They magnify your eyes—and your lines!—so you'll need a lighter makeup in softer, more subtle colors. Compensate for this magnification by having the lower part of your lenses tinted (see Choosing Tinted Lenses, p. 92)—not on a straight line but at a slight angle, about 45 degrees, from the inside bottom corner to the outside top corner. This works best on plastic lenses where color is painted on, not baked on, as it is with glass lenses. It should also be such a subtle tint that what's visible through the lens is merely the natural warmth of the skin.

If *you're nearsighted and wear bifocals*, your eye lines will be in double trouble: The top of the lenses will magnify your eyes, the bottom will minimize your eyes, so soft subtle makeup, especially for the cheeks, is more crucial than ever. Ruth Domber, a New York City optician and owner of 10/10 Optics, recommends tinted bifocals—they'll soften your lines plus mitigate the bifocal line. Or you could get "invisible bifocals" without any line at all.

If *you're farsighted*, your lenses make your eyes look larger, so you should wear stronger, darker (though never iridescent) makeup. Eyeliner is a must, as is extra concealer to make the whites of the eyes brighter. Use a dark shadow/highlighter under the brow as well as more color on the outer half of the eye. Two tips: (1) even though you're keeping your makeup dark, don't go to darker tinted lenses; and (2) if your farsightedness makes it difficult to see clearly enough to apply tidy makeup, invest in some very long handled brushes.

If *you're farsighted and wear bifocals*, you'll have more magnification and blurring so your makeup should be more defined (more so than if you were nearsighted), but not as dark as if you were just wearing a farsighted (non-bifocal) lens; and you should have tinted angles (as discussed above).

MORE EYE-LIFTS WITH GLASSES

Fitting the Frames

- Your glasses should never extend past your temporal jawbone line (the end of your face, see below, left), or the center of your face will cave in (if you're nearsighted) or your crow's-feet will be magnified (if you're farsighted).
- Consider your face shape: If you have an oval face, you can wear any frame; if you have a round face, go for any shape but round, which will make you look like an egg; if you have a square face, wear any shape but square, which will make you look like a box; if you have a heart-shape face, choose a frame with more "weight" on the bottom. And no matter what your face shape, never wear winged glasses that swerve at the temples or upside-down frames—both are unflattering. (See below, right.)
- Take your hairstyle into account, too: Generally speaking, a sleek cut looks best with biggish frames (see opposite); a fuller style with slimmer ones.

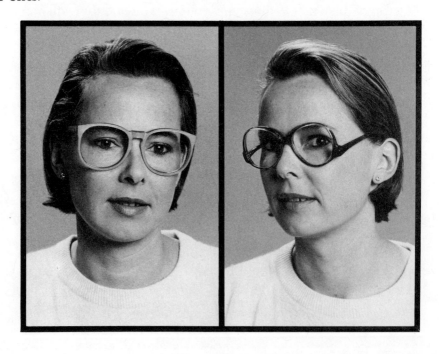

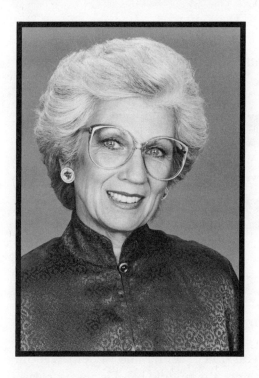

Picking Frame Color

Best colors for lined eyes: anything but flat gray, dark brown, bright red, blue-orange or Day-Glo • If you like metal frames, wear matte bronze or pewter, never gold or silver, which look like braces on the face • If you have wide-set eyes, go for colored frames; if you have close-set eyes, get a color-graduating frame with a shade that goes deeper toward the outer edges of the frame • Don't match frame color to eyeshadow, but don't choose contrasting or clashing colors either—orange frames with pink highlighter, for example • And never buy frames with initials.

A lot of women have a difficult time rationalizing spending $125–$150 for glasses. But, as Ruth Domber pointed out to me, you probably have several pairs of shoes. . . . What do people see first—and look at more—your feet or your face? Good point, I think.

Choosing Tinted Lenses

Ruth Domber places her customers into one of two color categories—blue or yellow—based on their hair color.

"Blue-lens" candidates have:	Best lens tints to hide wrinkles are:
ash, gray, dull brown or black hair with no yellow or gold	mauves, purples, pinks, lilacs—never yellow- or orange-based colors
"Yellow-lens" candidates have:	Best lens tints to hide wrinkles are:
reddish blond, golden, amber or chestnut hair	melon, pinky-peach, khaki, mustard, sand, rosy brown, turquoise, green, coral

Something to consider: gradient-tinted lenses, which Ruth says are one of the best ways to soften eye lines. They have three "color" bands. (I never even knew there was such a thing; you don't see the line of demarcation; neither do you see a "tinted" world, since the middle band is always clear!)

Best gradient tinted lenses for *a blue-lens candidate*: Top band is best-tint color (see chart, above) based on your eye shadow, not matched perfectly but one or two shades darker so the shadow color appears buffed and soft; the middle is clear and so makes eye whites brighter (don't ever get tinted lenses unless the middle, through which you look, is clear, or you could hurt your eyes); the bottom band should be a color "matched" to your blush (e.g., pink and mauve tones)—don't choose too dark a tint here because you don't want too much contrast between the lens and your cheek color.

Tip: Bring your makeup to your optician and show him the colors you want matched. Also, put smudges of eyeshadow and blusher on the order form so whoever is making up the lens will have a color reference.

For *yellow-lens candidates*: The top tint should be a shade or two darker than your best-tint color (see chart, above) based on your eye shadow color; the middle should be clear; and the bottom tint should be a sand or peach tone like your blush.

FACE MAKEUP: HOLDING BACK THE LINES

When you begin to age, three things happen to the skin on your face: It becomes thinner (because normal fat padding dissipates), less elastic (because the amount of collagen decreases) and paler (because it loses some of its pigment). Therefore, now's the time to learn how to use face makeup—foundation, blusher and powder—to your best advantage.

Foundation

CHOOSING THE RIGHT COLOR AND TEXTURE

- Select a light-textured foundation or a tinted moisturizer that'll let your skin show through. Heavy foundations make you look older, not better.
- Go for a color in the beige family—don't try to add color to your face with a peach or rose foundation. Let your blusher do that for you.
- You want a color that's as close to your natural skin tone as possible. Go darker only if you're tan. Whatever you do, do not choose a color that's darker than your natural skin color because you think it'll make you look tan—it'll just look unnatural and emphasize lines. Before you buy, test the color on your face—on, say, your cheek or forehead—and see if it blends into your skin; if it doesn't, it's the wrong color. Don't go by bottle color—it almost always looks darker than the foundation really is.
- If you have red wrinkles (broken capillaries), use a lavender corrector under your foundation.
- If you have deep laugh lines, use an emollient camouflage stick—two shades lighter than your foundation. Dot it on and blend. Follow with foundation.

HOW TO APPLY FOUNDATION

- The best way to smooth on foundation is with a slightly damp sponge—you'll get sheer, as well as even, coverage.
- Apply foundation only to your face—not to your neck or it'll seep into neck creases and get onto your clothes.

• After applying foundation, mist your face (a plant mister filled with tap water will do the trick). This will help set the makeup, give you a dewy finish.

How to Make Up for Period Problems

About five days before your period starts, hormonal changes can trigger increased oil production by the skin. When these oils mix with cosmetics, they often result in skin discoloration, exacerbated sometimes by the combined secretions of fatty acids, amino acids and eliminated toxins.

Rx: Before you apply your makeup, use a skin corrector that'll keep the sallow sebum color from altering the color of your foundation—light green usually works well. If you find that the increased oil activity makes your face shine, try dipping cotton in cold water and gently patting over your made-up face; follow with gentle patting with a piece of dry cotton. If need be, a quick dusting of translucent powder will help degleam, too.

> A good idea for when you need an extra lift, say after a long, tiring day: Apply a very thin film of any clear tightening mask to your face (avoiding the undereye area), allow it to dry and then smooth on your foundation.

Blusher

CHOOSING THE RIGHT COLOR

Use your hair color as a guide for selecting your cheek color. Use only matte-finish colors—the metallic flecks in iridescent ones will settle in the creases of your skin.

• If you're *blond*, use light tawny tones.
• If you're a *redhead*, go for peach and coral tones.
• If you're a *brunette*, choose rose, mauve or brown-red tones.
• If you're *gray*, try clear rose and red tones.

WHERE TO APPLY BLUSHER

Cheek-color belongs on your cheeks. Don't try to create cheekbones where they don't exist—you'll only create an unnatural, unflattering look. Here's how to find your cheeks and give them color.

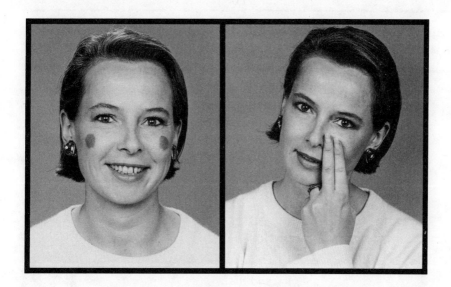

1. Smile into a mirror—you'll see where your cheeks are instantly.
2. Next, take two fingers and place them alongside your nose. The finger furthest from your nose is where blusher should begin.
3. Extend blush up and out toward the hairline at the temples to visually pull up your face. *Note:* Always stroke blusher on in an upward motion to "lift."

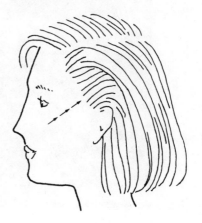

Margaret A. Hinders

Or just use your own natural glow as a guide. Here's a good way to boost circulation and bring a wonderful warm glow to your cheeks: Before you do your makeup, lie on a slantboard (or use an ironing board propped up on books on one end) for five to thirty minutes; you'll not only look fresher, you'll feel it, too.

> An easy do-it-yourself "chin lift"—brush on a deep mauve blush along the jawline from one ear to the other under the chin (see above).

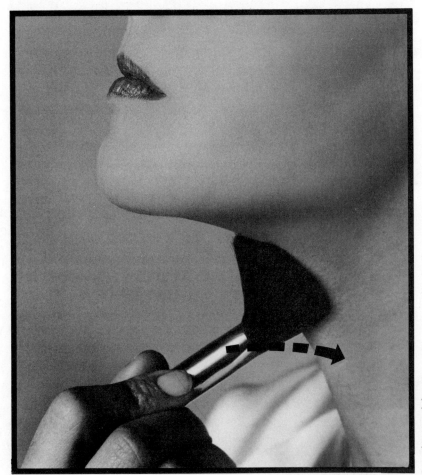

Dorothy Handelman

REAL-LIFE MAKEOVERS: TURN-BACK-THE-CLOCK TECHNIQUES

Here's all the proof you need that the right makeup colors used the right way—plus some simple hair styling and coloring—can literally take years off your looks. The six women here are not models . . . they're not actresses or celebrities; they're real women—just normal people like you and me. I think some of the tips we gave them may work wonders on you, too. For all the details see pages 101–08.

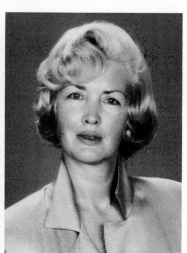

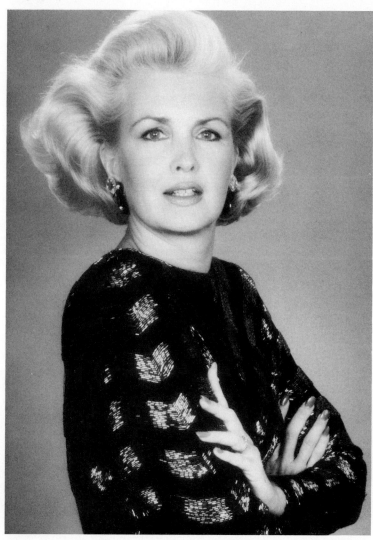

Evening dress by Fabrice

Blond and Beautiful

Barbara Alexis, forty-eight, looks at least ten years younger with stronger, brighter makeup colors and a fuller, more modern hairstyle.

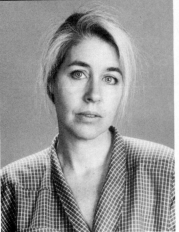

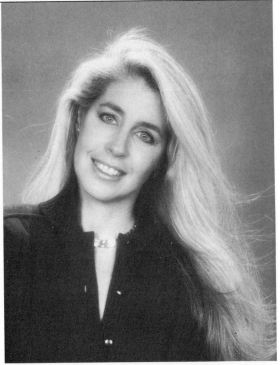

Rule-Breaking Beauty

Don't assume that long hair is aging! There are always exceptions to rules, as you can see on Bonnie Cantor, forty-five.

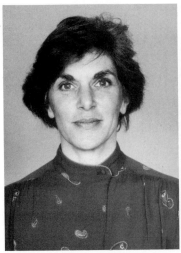

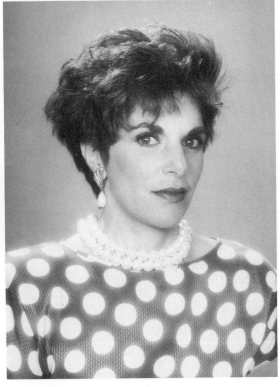

More Makeup, a More Natural Look

Deep earth tones applied carefully not only enhance the natural look on Jane Kauffmann, forty-four, they make it prettier, too.

Blouse by Ungaro

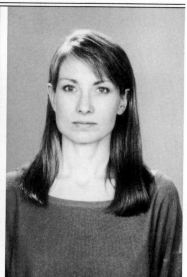

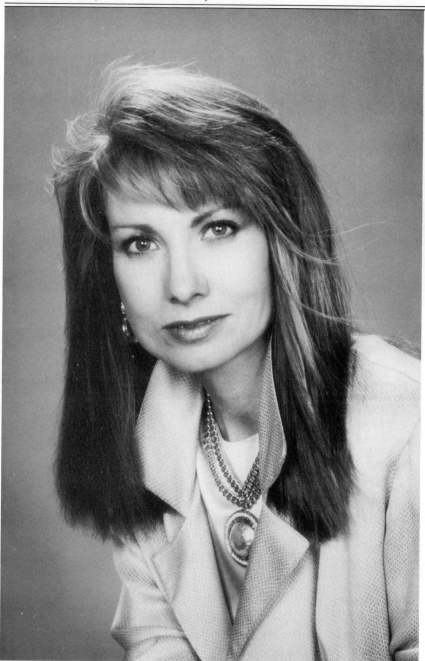

Youth-Enhancing Hair and Makeup

What Susan Reed, thirty-seven, needed was a little perking up: highlights in her hair, now starting to dull; and neutral, light-textured makeup to brighten and accentuate her features and to detract from the fine lines beginning to form.

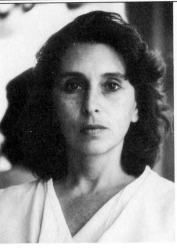

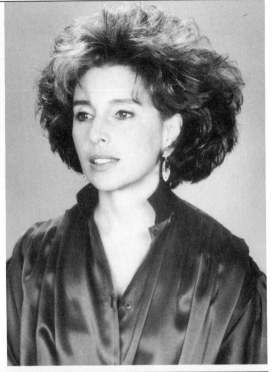

Blouse by Andre Van Pier

Antiaging Colors

Sun-damaged skin doesn't have to look old. Brighter makeup colors as well as brighter hair newly styled for maximum volume prove the point on Arlene Oxman, thirty-nine.

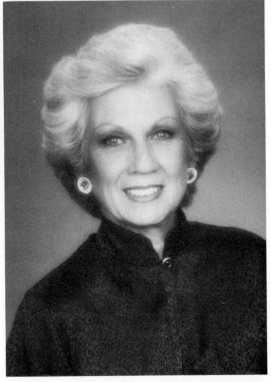

Gray and Gorgeous

On Kitty Tananbaum, fifty-seven, the brighter the gray the younger she looks. We brightened it, then applied her makeup in light, bright (but not harsh) colors.

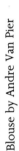

WHAT MADE UP THE REAL-LIFE MAKEOVERS

Barbara Alexis

It was hairstylist Garren who suggested we do a makeover on Barbara Alexis (who's on our cover). She's top model Kim Alexis's mother—and a real beauty in her own right, too.

As soon as Catherine and I saw Barbara we knew Garren had a good idea. She's as beautiful for her age as Kim is for hers—Barbara is forty-eight—and though she had her hair professionally cut and colored and knew something about makeup, her choices about both hair and makeup weren't, on most counts, working to her best advantage.

A lot of women with Barbara's blond hair would look old, but that's not what was making her older-looking: What aged her was her hairstyle. So Garren gave her a new, more modern cut with height and width that lifts her whole face . . . and makeup artist Sandy Linter taught her how to use a whole new palette of slightly stronger, brighter (but not harsh or garish) makeup colors, which flatter as they de-age.

On the Cover:

- Sandy applied a base to eyelids, lightening them, making them smooth and receptive to makeup.
- Next: She used a pencil, then a shadow to shape and color Barbara's eyes. Sandy used a gray pencil under her eyes and to line upper lids, blended it well and went over it all with gray shadow, also blended well.
- Over the gray, lavender shadow was feathered under the brow, in the crease and under the lower outer corner of the eye. (Sandy feels it's aging to use only one shade on the eye.)

> *Tip:* Consider applying eye makeup before face makeup—eyes are messier to do, but simple to clean up, especially if you don't have to worry about ruining your base or blusher.

- The finish: black mascara.
- Sandy used a Q-Tip to dab on foundation and a sponge to blend it against the grain of the skin "so it doesn't fall into the lines."
- For cheek contouring Sandy used a small amount of rosy pink blush.
- Rose lipstick, the same tone as the blusher, completes the look.

In the Makeover Section:

- For an all-out glamorous evening, deeper colors were added so Barbara's look wouldn't fade into the night light or pale against the brightness of her dress.
- Under lower lashes, voilet shadow.
- Hot pink shadow was brushed on under brows.
- To define eyes, very dark brown liquid liner went along lash line.
- Hot pink lipstick gave lips a hot, sexy look.

Bonnie Cantor

On a recent trip to Canyon Ranch Spa in Tucson, Arizona, Catherine and I noticed Bonnie right away: She looked great in her leotard, with her hair pulled straight back and no makeup whatsoever. Were we surprised to learn that she was in her forties (forty-five, to be exact)! We saw only a few flaws—and we knew that just a little makeup and hair fixing could work wonders on them.

We didn't change the length of her hair; nor did we want to change the highlights she'd already had put into her hair. (Though it's generally aging for a woman over forty to have below-shoulder-length hair, for Bonnie it's her long hair that makes her look younger than her years.) All we did: curl her hair with a curling iron to give it body and make it smooth and healthy-looking too.

What we did change, though, was Bonnie's no-makeup look. We gave Bonnie a basic makeup that enhances her healthy good looks; it's a very youthful look created with natural, earth-tone colors. The point: Many women (Bonnie included) think makeup will give them a made-up look; wrong, as you can see from Francois's makeup.

- First, Francois bleached Bonnie's brows, which were too dark against her pale complexion and so heavy they closed in the eye area.
- A moisturizer was smoothed on her face.
- Francois began eyes with a black liner as close as he could get to upper lashes.
- With the same brush and same color, Francois applied a soft shadowline under lower lashes. He brushed the lids with a light amount of translucent powder to smooth and even out the skin tone.
- Next, mascara.
- Then Francois applied a warm brown shadow to the browbone area to eliminate the puffiness most women have at this age.
- Beige shadow evened out the skin tone on the eyelid.
- A creamy beige base minimized veins under the eyes.
- A slightly darker base was used to even out pigmentations on the neck, right under the chin to shorten her nose, and under the lower lip to create a curve there.
- A dusting of loose translucent powder sealed the makeup on face and neck.
- A golden color powder (also translucent) went on cheeks.
- More loose translucent powder was dusted all over as a final face polish.
- Lips were lined in soft mauve, which was then blended onto lip with a brush.
- Cheek gel in pink was applied to lips as a stain.
- Then a lip balm was smoothed onto lips to condition them and seal in color. *Tip:* The reason you should use the balm before the gel is that if you do the opposite, the color will stick to the balm, not your lips.

Jane Kauffmann

Catherine met Jane skiing in Taos one Christmas, and when she learned that Jane was forty-four, she was immediately impressed with how young she looked—at least under her ski hat: She had the most wonderful natural look. Then one night Jane invited Catherine to a party: "I was shocked when I saw her 'dressed.'"

What Catherine couldn't see under Jane's ski hat was a salt-and-pepper hair color that drained Jane's healthy-looking complexion of all its color. So the first thing we did was send Jane to hair colorist Louis Licari, who removed the gray with a semipermanent color, making it all one dark color, and then used a permanent color to create highlights around the sides and front to enhance skin color.

Next stop was hairstylist Gad Cohen: He cut the sides to emphasize the width on either side of her face, which is long and narrow, and he layered the top, removing weight from both sides of the part so that she'd no longer have a definite part. Gad also removed "weight" near the nape but left length "to keep the style feminine." In front, he cut bangs in a C shape around each eye so Jane's almond-shaped eyes would stand out. To style he used mousse only on the roots for a spiky, full look.

Finally, a whole new makeup: Jane rarely wore any makeup at all, thinking that was the way to enhance her natural look. We convinced her otherwise. Here's Craig Gadson's step-by-step application for a natural but dramatic new look.

- Since Jane doesn't have a lot of space for color between her lashes and brows, Craig curled lashes carefully: "When lashes are properly curled you can use less eye makeup," he says.
- Inside the rim of the upper lid, Craig used a very dark brown eyeliner, which defines the eye without being obvious.
- On the inside of the lower lid, Craig used a charcoal-gray liner.
- He applied a brownish-copper shadow to lids, a matte beige highlighter under the brows and one coat of mascara to the lashes.
- To tone down the red in Jane's cheeks, Craig used a green color corrector.
- He then applied foundation in a shade that matched her skin color, mixing it with a spritz of mineral water to make it sheerer on her oily skin.
- Under Jane's eyes, instead of a concealer, which he feels tends to "separate and crease," Craig used a base a shade lighter than her foundation.
- On cheeks, he used a rosy pink blush.
- To balance strong eyes, Craig used rose-colored lip liner and a matching lipstick with just a hint of gloss on the bottom lip.

Susan Reed

Susan is a natural beauty and—at thirty-seven—suffers from the same problem a lot of beautiful women suffer from as they get older: When they need to change their no-makeup look to one that enhances and makes them look younger, they're not used to taking the time it takes—and they don't know exactly what to do.

First her hair, always long and gorgeous, is now a little duller in color. We sent Susan to Louis Licari, who brightened it in varying light shades, especially around the face. Next stop was Gad Cohen, who changed the long straight-across bangs, which at one time made her look younger but were now pulling her face down, making her look older than her years. He beveled the hair around her face, removing the bulk on top and cut bangs with points that gave a sparser, lighter feeling. Last, he "slide-cut" the sides to give the illusion of layers.

Since Susan has such fine features and pale skin, Craig Gadson gave her a neutral light-textured makeup that enhanced her good looks (bright bold colors would age her dramatically).

- A spritzing of mineral water and a fine layer of moisturizer smoothed Susan's skin and helped foundation go on evenly.
- On upper lids, Craig used a charcoal liner, which he smudged for softness with a Q-Tip. Over charcoal liner, he used a medium blue liner and blended it with a sponge-tip applicator. The same medium blue was used to make a fine unblended line.
- Then Craig used a violet eye shadow, dark at the outer corner, lighter in the crease, blending to pale pink shadow in the middle of the lid.
- A gray pencil on the outer corner of the lid was blended up into the crease.
- On browbone: a highlighter in pale peach.
- Craig curled Susan's lashes and used black mascara generously.
- Now, foundation, the same as the one used on eyelids, and a dab of concealer under the eyes.
- To set the foundation, translucent powder dusted on with a big fluffy brush.
- Pink blush accented Susan's high cheekbones.
- Lips were outlined with a taupe pencil, filled in with a matching lipstick.

Arlene Oxman

Arlene has beautiful, unusual features and a wonderful olive complexion. But after spending summer after summer in the sun without any protection—she, like so many women, opted for a tan instead of a wrinkle-free face—at thirty-nine she is prematurely lined. Arlene is a prime example of what proper hair coloring, a good cut and a well-thought-out makeup can do to improve sun-damaged skin.

The hair coloring: For the past few years Arlene had been coloring her hair with either a henna or a one-color semipermanent coloring. The result in both cases: too flat—and aging—a shade. So we sent her to Louis Licari, who used varying shades of highlights, especially around the face, that work to soften her lines.

The cut: Arlene's long, layered, almost shaglike haircut dragged her face down and made her look older than she was. "It was totally the wrong shape for her heart-shaped face," says Garren, who shortened it in back to give it more body and fullness. He cut a fringe bang in front and layered the top short to accentuate her eyes, the focal point of her face. To style, he used lots of mousse, scrunching hair and fluffing it up as it dried naturally.

The makeup: Just as the brighter hair color applied by Louis compensated for Arlene's sun-damaged skin, so, too, do Sandy Linter's brighter makeup colors.

- To instantly lift her eyes, create more of an arch, Sandy tweezed the brows and used a brow pencil to fill in where brows had become sparse.
- Matte purple (bright but not dark) pencil liner was used on outer half of lid and along lash line. With a brush, Sandy blended the purple pencil well. Tip: Because Arlene has naturally deep-set eyes, Sandy was careful not to line the entire eye, which would only make eyes recede further.
- Bright purple shadow was brushed over the pencil to soften the line.
- Over the upper lid and onto the brow a peach shadow was applied.
- Foundation was smoothed on with a damp sponge. Under Arlene's eyes where there are wrinkles, Sandy blended against the grain of the skin so the foundation wouldn't settle into the creases.

- To blend dark sunspots into the rest of Arlene's face, Sandy used a foundation in a shade darker than her natural skin tone.
- Under eyes, in the center of the nose and across the forehead, a dusting of translucent powder eliminated shine.
- Matte pink blusher highlighted cheekbones. *Tip: Don't put your blusher on under your cheekbones or you'll create a gaunt "old" look.*
- A touch of yellow shadow went right under outer corners of the brow to bring out the yellow in Arlene's eyes.
- Lips were lined with skin-tone mauve and were filled in with bright coral.

Kitty Tananbaum

She looks good for her age—she's fifty-seven—but when Catherine and I first met her we could see immediately that with the right haircolor and cut and the proper makeup she could look even better.

Kitty's an exception to a lot of rules. At first glance, your immediate reaction is that she ought to cut her hair short and color her gray hair dark. But on reconsideration you see that with her skin tone and face shape neither is appropriate. What Kitty needed was a brightening of the gray—a dramatic dark color change would be too harsh next to her pale porcelain skin. On her, gray looks special, even youthful! And because her face is full, it would have been too aging to cut her hair too close to her ears, a mistake a lot of women make when they are in their mid-fifties. It's simply too dramatic—and unflattering—a look.

After colorist Cida Nery brightened the gray and stylist Aldo Giacomello curled and combed it for added volume, Pablo Manzoni gave her subtle (de-aging) makeup.

- Pablo first used a lot of freshener to tighten pores. He followed up with a regular moisturizer, then an opaque white-colored moisturizer to give skin a luminescence.
- To begin eyes, Pablo used an eye makeup base that works to "keep eye shadow from creasing in already-creased lids."
- To enhance her blue eyes, a blue-hyacinth cream shadow was blended with a brush on the lid. *Tip: It's best for women with small lids to keep*

their makeup mirror below their chins so they look down into it . . . and the whole lid shows so they can count on even coverage.

- A dark gray liquid liner was used to rim the outer half of the upper lid, and, before it dried, Pablo smudged it with a moist brush to soften the edges: "Liner should not look like a line . . . but the root of the lashes."
- A silver-fox cream shadow was smoothed on under lower lid as a liner.
- Right over it, a powder pencil in periwinkle applied lightly makes the faintest shadow of a line, and dark blue liner in the inner rim of the lower lashes instantly brightens eyes.
- Black mascara was applied to upper lashes, first from the top, then from the underside, combed after every coating; ditto on lower lashes.
- On eyebrows Pablo drew hairlines with a cake-brown liner and fine brush to fill in where Kitty's brows had thinned.
- After cleaning up the eye area, Pablo blended a base "to a great extent" with a sponge.
- A wine cream rouge was applied high on cheekbones, close to the eyes to brighten eyes as well as to highlight cheeks.
- A matte sheer colorless face powder was dusted on all over to set the foundation.
- Pablo uses layers of blusher to make color last longer. Antique-rose powder blusher ("a marvelous color for women with gray hair") was used over the cream rouge on cheeks and cheekbones way up to the outer corner of the eyes. The same powder blush was also dusted on the temples to give an all-over healthy glow. Be careful it doesn't get on white hair!
- Lips were lined and colored with a pink pencil: "Lip pencil doesn't bleed like lipstick does," says Pablo, who smoothed on fuchsia lipstick over it.

FACE MAKEUP, PART II

Powder

No matter what your skin tone, use only a fine-textured, matte-finish translucent powder—no sparkle or color, which will only call attention to fine lines and wrinkles. Both Catherine and I prefer loose to compact powder because it goes on more evenly and lighter. This is our preference; it may not be yours. . . . With a large fluffy brush or cotton puff, apply only a light dusting of powder (on superoily skin you may find cotton balls work best). *Note:* If your skin tends to be dry, stay away from powder—it will only make it look drier . . . and older.

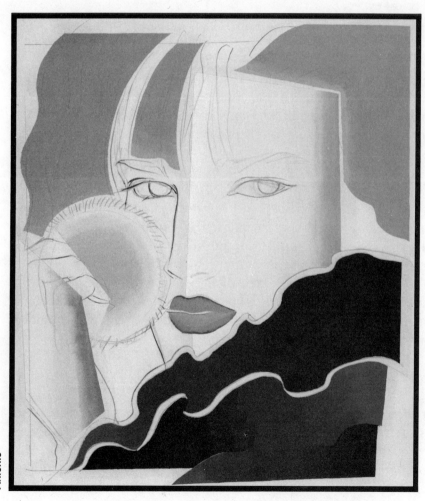

Antonio

Here's *how to apply powder* so it doesn't collect in lines: Dip brush or puff into loose powder you've put into the palm of your hand (you'll get less than if you dip it right into the container, and it's always easier to add powder than to subtract it). Shake or blow excess off brush and start at your chin, dusting up over your nose. When you get to the top of forehead, turn the puff over and dust across forehead, down each cheek to jaw and chin. To finish, use a large fluffy makeup brush to whisk away excess.

Tip: If you use pressed powder and it's collecting in creases, it's because you're letting it sit on surface of skin. To do correctly: With a sponge, press the powder into the foundation so it holds onto the base and doesn't look powdery or cakey.

LIPS

You've heard of lips bleeding—that doesn't always mean they're sore, chapped and bloody. What it does mean is that fine lines have formed around the lips into which lipstick seeps or "bleeds." But with the right lipstick and the proper application, you can avoid this problem altogether.

Lip Liner

As you age, your natural lip line becomes less defined, and lip liner becomes more important, not only to add definition to the shape of your mouth but to keep lip color in place, keep it from bleeding. To apply: Using a matte pencil liner in a soft rose color (avoid colors that are too brown), outline your natural lip line with a thick line. Soften with your finger or cotton-tip applicator and get ready to fill in with lip color. If you have trouble keeping the line straight, stretch your lip over your teeth with your middle and index fingers on either side of your mouth.

Lipstick

Lip color should be the same color as the liner; you should not be able to distinguish between the two. Choose a cream formula with a semimatte finish in clean, warm colors like mauve, peach, rose, coral; stay away from colors that are too white (pastels with a white base), too dark (deep burgundies) or too bright (fire engine red); they'll just call attention to wrinkles around the mouth. (*Important:* Keep your lip color in the same color family as your blusher.)

Tips to keep lip color in place: Apply foundation to your lips, let dry, then line and fill in with lipstick. You can use lip liner instead of lipstick: Line lips, fill in with liner and apply a tiny amount of clear gloss over it. If you have deep vertical lip lines, don't use lip gloss—it will run into the lines around lips.

To lift a droopy mouth: If the corners of your lips have begun to droop, don't apply lipstick all the way to the corners; stop short. It's not noticeable and it's a good trick to uplift lips visually. Lift lip liner very slightly where you stop short, and use a darker lip color on the bottom lip than on the top lip.

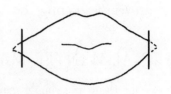

Margaret A. Hinders

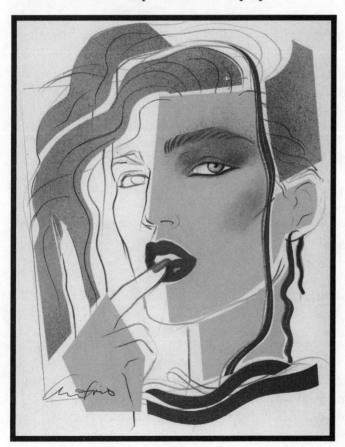

To detract from upper lip lines: Use gloss and use it only in the middle of the bottom lip.

Three tips to keep lips smooth, wrinkle-free:

1. Simply brush lips with a toothbrush you've softened in hot water. Pat on a lip emollient. Wipe gently.
2. On lines around your mouth, use an exfoliator in a cream base. Wipe off and gently smooth on a moisturizer.
3. Use a lip repair product to hydrate skin, fill in lines and cracks and prevent feathering, too.

SPECIAL WINTER MAKEUP PRECAUTIONS

- Just as I said you should make sure you're using oil-based creams in winter, I also suggest you use an oil-based foundation in winter. And choose a foundation with a little pink in it during the months when your complexion pales and looks slightly sallow.
- This bears repeating, too: Choose a foundation (and a lipstick) that has an SPF of at least 4. It's better to be safe than sorry!
- Cream rouges and eye shadows are better choices than powder blushes and powder shadows in winter—they offer more protection.

SPECIAL SUMMER MAKEUP PRECAUTIONS

- After sun exposure, when skin has thickened, go for a light-textured foundation. Your heavier winter one will look too unnatural.

  Tip: Lighten an already light textured foundation—or your heavier winter one—by applying your foundation while your moisturizer is still damp; it'll allow the color to glide on smoothly, evenly . . . sheerly!

CLOTHES CONSCIOUSNESS

Like makeup, clothes and accessories should be chosen carefully to detract from wrinkles . . . or they'll accentuate your lines and you (and everyone else, too, for that matter) will really understand what the cliché "you are what you wear" means. And you won't like it.

To get all the dos and don'ts, I called Christine Kunzelman, who owns the Panache Appearance Studios in Torrance, California. She caters to housewives and career women, giving total appearance makeovers that include every-thing from skin, hair and makeup to figure analysis and fashion consulting.

Color

Do choose soft, subdued colors like peach or pink that'll tone down every-thing, including wrinkles.

Don't wear bold bright colors next to the face—they'll draw too much attention to wrinkles.

Don't wear black without adding a necklace of colored stones or gold to offset the starkness against wrinkled skin.

Prints

Do stick to small prints or, better yet, solids, which are good un-busy "frames" for the face.

Don't wear big bold prints next to your face—and stay away from lots of lace at the face: Although it's very feminine, in combination with wrinkles, it denotes older rather than younger—the contrast between little-girl frilly and older skin is too severe.

Necklines

Do choose blouses and dresses with high collars, and soft bows that cover turkey necks and/or distract the eye from wrinkles. If you don't have the problem of a lined neck, soft open collars can be very pretty, as they'll draw the eye down, away from the face.

Don't choose plunging V-necks or large scoop necklines. Pleated collars, like lace, put too many frills near the face.

Necklaces

Do make sure that whatever necklace you wear doesn't clasp the neck and pull on your skin. If it's big and bulky and/or busy, make sure it is long to draw attention down and away from a wrinkled neck and/or face. Pearls, a good-looking gold chain or collarlike necklace that sits on your collarbones are good choices.

Don't wear chokers—they cause the neck to wrinkle even if it hasn't—or anything else around your neck that will cause pleating of neck skin when you move your head. Never tie a scarf under the chin—it will accent sagging jowls.

Earrings

Do stick to clip-on earrings worn close to the face.

Don't wear long dangling earrings that tug on your earlobes and make them look longer, stretched-out and older (plus they can draw the whole face down). Lots of glitter will call attention to crow's-feet and laugh lines.

Rings/Bracelets

Do wear only small, simple band-styled rings, a lightweight unflashy bracelet or delicate watch.

Don't wear heavy, ornate rings or a wristful of bracelets if your hands are wrinkled or have a lot of brown spots.

FIVE

WRINKLE-REMOVING

HAIR COLORING

AND STYLING

You might wonder why in a book about wrinkles there's a whole chapter on hair. In a nutshell: Hair, like makeup, can be an effective line hider. The right hair color and style can mean the difference between looking great and looking tired, haggard—and old!

Before I get to the specifics on coloring and styling, I want to make one thing clear: Hair, like skin, ages. And like skin, too, it ages gradually (from about eighteen on), though most women don't realize it because they're generally too busy worrying about their skin. All of a sudden one morning they wake up and their hair looks old!

Basically, there are three main factors that make hair old-looking. It *dries out, dulls,* mainly because of years of abuse, particularly chemical processing; *grays* because less pigment is being formed; and *thins* as a natural result of aging and/or because of poor diet, illness, stress, certain medications, too-tight curlers, too stiff a hairbrush, overbrushing and/or overprocessing. With creative coloring and styling you can not only camouflage your hair's age, but yours, too!

HOW TO COLOR YOUR HAIR (AND YOUR FACE!) YOUNG

Think of hair color the way you do makeup: "Like makeup, hair color is a necessity, not a luxury, for women who are getting older," says Louis Licari, color director at La Coupe Salon in New York City and author of *Color Your Life . . . With Haircolor* (Putnam,1985). "You can use color to deemphasize your wrinkled or sagging skin," he says. "Plus it can improve hair texture and boost its body and shine." Two examples:

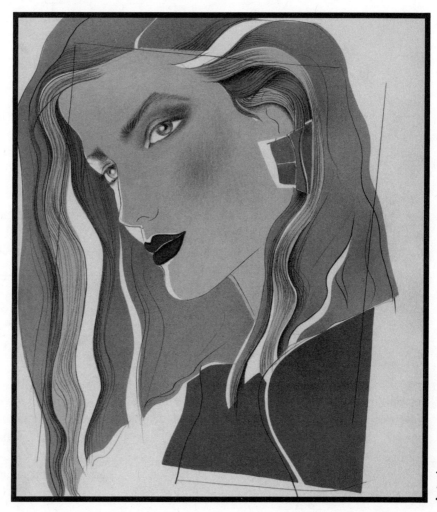

Antonio

To uplift droopy eyes, add sparkle: Louis puts a few bright highlights on the hair right above each eye . . . and he suggests lightening eyebrows, too, if they're so dark they contribute to the heavy look. (See opposite.)

To minimize a double chin, focus attention up to eyes: Louis uses highlights just on the top section of the hair to focus the eye up. In addition, he recommends a chin-length blunt cut—again, so lightness is up top. (See below.)

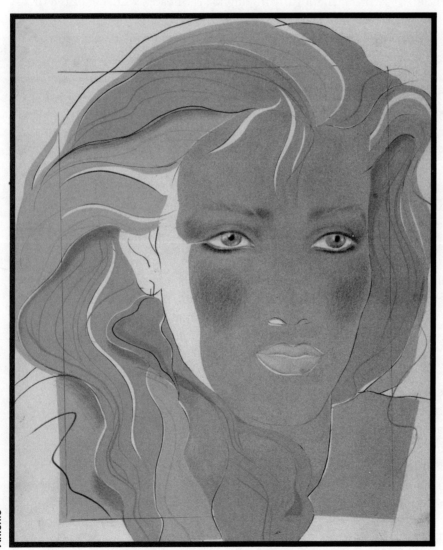

Antonio

Basically, there are three main categories of hair color:

- *Permanent color* can lighten or darken hair, cover gray or enhance a color by matching it. It lasts until hair grows out.

  Highlighting falls into this category: Properly chosen, highlights are always right—if you're blond, you need contrasting shades of blond (to keep hair from looking bleached); brunettes look best with deep golden brown and mahogany highlights; redheads, whose hair is a mix of beige, yellow-red and dark brown, need highlights of any other color (or their hair can take on an unmistakable dullness).

- *Semipermanent color* can darken hair, create highlights or cover gray (it can't lighten because it contains no peroxide). It lasts through several shampoos.

- *Temporary color* can enhance your natural color, add shine and cover gray, but it can't lighten your hair. It lasts through only one shampoo.

  Two temporary rinses from Louis that you can make yourself: *To brighten blond hair,* steep ¼ cup chamomile tea in a quart of boiling water, strain, cool and rinse through hair after shampooing (don't rinse off). *To brighten brunet hair,* steep 1 tablespoon rosemary in 1 pint of boiling water, strain, cool and rinse through hair after shampooing (don't rinse off).

Which type of color you choose is really a matter of personal preference. If you've never colored your hair before, consider experimenting with semipermanent or temporary color before you settle on a permanent one. Another idea for the more cautious: Before you plunge into something permanent, try on wigs.

After you settle on the type of color, you'll have to decide which shade to use: whether you should go lighter, darker, cover gray or just highlight your natural color. My feeling is that you should always stick as close to your natural color as possible. I think that in almost every case women look best when they don't try to buck what Mother Nature intended for them. Too dramatic and/or extreme a change—say, hair that's too black (it creates shadows on the face), too blond (it drains color) or is frosted (it's too harsh and garish-looking)—is guaranteed to accentuate every flaw and add years to your looks. Tip: Never, ever go for dense all-over color—remember, natural hair is a blend of colors.

> If you change your hair color, change your makeup, too—it casts a different shadow on your face, making your skin tone change, too.

When in doubt, it's usually a wise choice to go lighter rather than darker because brightness tends to make skin glow, look younger. The only exception would be if you have very fine hair. Light makes very fine light-colored hair look finer and thinner; you may be best off with just a few warm highlights around your face.

TO GRAY OR NOT TO GRAY?

That's the question most women have to face at one time or another, and it's a big one. Whatever age gray strikes—some spot gray in their twenties, others in their thirties . . . and almost all by the time they reach their forties— it connotes aging, and most women panic. Don't panic (and don't pull out gray strands, either—they'll still grow back gray, but coarser, kinkier). You may just like your gray (it looks great on some women), but if you don't you can cover it—easily.

If You Opt to Stay Gray

Gray hair looks best if you're blue-eyed and/or fair-skinned. It actually can add softness to your face that may take years off your looks. Louis suggests a diluted bluing rinse (half rinse, half water for half the suggested time) to keep all-gray hair light and bright, and to take away yellow cast. Also, if you do decide to stay gray, realize that whatever you do to your hair—curl it, cut it, perm it—it will stand out more and enhance the lines you have. The reason, once again: Light hair reflects light to make everything more pronounced. (A word of caution: Be extra careful perming gray hair, because the lack of melanin causes perms to under- or overprocess.) So go easy on gray hair. And, in my opinion, a style that's neither too long nor too short is best.

Tip: If you're dark eyed and/or olive skinned, the salt-and-pepper stage of graying creates a contrast that is often too intense and aging with your dark complexion, and you'll need to color it.

Gray hair is hair without pigment. Actually it's pure white, but next to your natural color it looks gray, hence the misnomer.

If You Hate Your Gray

Before you do anything, make sure you avoid these common (and blatantly aging) mistakes:

- Don't think you have to go dark to cover gray—you could end up with a drab, dull head of hair.
- Don't think ash blond frosting is your best bet for camouflaging gray— the ash tones will make your gray look grayer.
- Don't just go back to your original color—it may not be right for you anymore (remember your skin tone has changed—aged!—too).

Here, three simple solutions to getting rid of gray:

1. If you're just beginning to find a few gray strands here and there, use a temporary rinse a shade darker than your natural color. Or if you're in need of a touch-up and only have a minute to do it, try these quick color fixes: Use your mascara to cover gray by brushing the wand over the gray hairs; use the new color mousses in dark colors like burgundy or brown; or use one of the new no-peroxide hair glosses.
2. After a more permanent answer? Semipermanent color will cover gray strands and blend them into your natural color; and, in fact, in addition to actually softening the hair itself and adding shine, it can turn gray hair strands into very natural highlights. If you only have a bit of gray, choose a semipermanent color in an apricot-blond shade. Louis told me that often the gray hair that first appears (usually right around the face) is often the best to highlight . . . as long as (a) you never apply the color all the way to the scalp because new growth will show, and (b) you leave a few strands of gray for a natural look.
3. If your hair is more than 50 percent gray and you want to cover your gray completely, permanent color will do the job best.

BODY BUILDERS FOR FINE AND/OR THIN HAIR

While there is almost nothing more youthful than a full, glorious head of hair, there is almost nothing (not even wrinkles—just ask any man who is beginning to lose his hair) more aging than fine and/or thin hair.

There's a lot of confusion about fine and thin hair. The first point to note is that there is, indeed, a difference between the two: *Fine* refers to the diameter of each strand (it's so small the hair bends easily, is limp and droopy). Thin refers to the number of strands on your head, a number that usually decreases with age (while you may have 700 hairs per square centimeter at age twenty, you'll only have 500 when you're fifty) and seems to become apparent overnight (up to 50 percent of the hair can be lost before you notice it). Whichever you have, the effect is the same: Your fine and/or thin hair is adding years to your looks.

Anyone with thinning hair should consult a dermatologist, who can either help you quell temporary thinning or assure you that your hair's thinning is just a natural evolution, the result of heredity and age. And in cases in which thinning actually becomes severe hair loss (called female pattern baldness, or FPB), a doctor can prescribe certain medications, which won't necessarily promote regrowth but will definitely prevent further loss.

There's a relatively new drug that more and more physicians are using to combat thinning hair: Minoxidil. It has been shown to work. A friend of ours, in fact, uses the lotion religiously and has a whole new head of hair. Of course, there's the transplant option, too—the punch graft method—but this requires three days of bandages, a month of having transplanted hairs visible and two to three more months before permanent growth begins.

In addition to these medical "cures" for thinning hair, there are many other ways to boost thin hair's body, too—and they work for fine hair as well.

Care

Dirt and oil can weigh down fine and/or thin hair, so a good shampoo is of the utmost importance, as is a postshampoo conditioner, which will keep static electricity in check—fine/thin hair is more susceptible to static electricity and becomes flyaway because it has less weight to keep it down.

Tip: If your hair falls flat, you may be using too heavy a conditioner; switch to something lighter or oil free.

Cut

Keep it short (shorter even than chin length if you can; no longer than shoulder length) because the longer the hair, the heavier it is and the limper it'll hang. Go for layers, which lighten the load, and consider, too, short underlayers, which will help support the longer layers over them.

Coloring/Perming

Coloring swells the hairshaft and then seals it, making hair heavier and more controllable. Plus, it can go a long way toward visually thickening hair, too. Remember, very light hair looks transparent; so if you darken it, it will obviously look less so—and thicker.

Perms and body waves, by definition, add volume. You can blow-dry permed hair to fluff it up even more . . . or you can combine a layered cut with a body wave for a modern, full look.

Styling

Blow-drying is one sure way to add volume to fine and/or thin hair that's medium length or longer. How to: Bend over and blow your hair in an upside-down position; to prevent damage stop while your hair is still a little damp. Note: It's not the heat that adds body but the air stream. (This doesn't mean, though, that you should use a blow dryer just on a cool setting—the low-heat settings are to hold a curl once hair has been styled.)

Warning: Keep the dryer from blowing on your face. The hot air will dry out your skin.

Mousses are wonderful body builders for fine and/or thin hair because they add body and shine without any stickiness or stiffness. Gad Cohen, a New York City stylist and owner of the Gad Salon, taught Catherine, who has baby-fine hair, how to use mousse to get more body: Apply it right from the nozzle. Catherine takes the nozzle and "mousses" her scalp in neat little partlike rows. (See opposite.) With the pads of her fingers, she massages the scalp, creating friction and roughing up (the operative words) the roots. As it dries, she massages more and scrunches the ends with her fingers for a full, tousled look she said she once thought was an impossibility for her unless she wore a wig. To finish: She finger combs, being careful not to pull her fingers all the way through to the ends—doing so could pull out body.

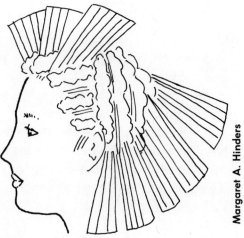

Margaret A. Hinders

Another way to use mousse to lift fine and/or thin hair away from the face: After you mousse, comb hair back, tie a ribbon around your head so it's about 2 inches from the hairline (or use 3-inch combs) and push it forward to puff the front. Let dry.

Hairsprays aren't just for holding power anymore; used the right way, they can give the same kind of lift as mousses and, in fact, are a little stronger than mousses (so they can work for medium-thick hair as well as fine-to-medium hair). Without even wetting your hair, you can spritz a hairspray on at the roots for a quick lift and blow it dry (just hold the dryer so it blows hair up from the scalp and away from the face).

One thing I recently learned from Garren, a top New York City hairstylist, is that you can use spray in conjunction with mousse for all-over body that really holds. This technique works wonders on fine and/or thin hair: After you apply mousse and it begins to dry, bend over and spray the underside of your hair, flip it back and spray the topside. Again, use the pads of your fingers to lift the roots of your hair and scrunch. When hair is completely dry, finger comb—and spray once more for hold.

> **Best way to revive a style you've created with mousses or sprays: Just spritz with water!**

WRINKLE-REMOVING HAIRSTYLES

On the next six pages you'll find de-aging hairstyles that are modern and up-to-date—and classic enough to cut across all age lines. They'll work for almost every woman, every look. Of course, you can experiment and vary the style to suit your personal style, too, but stick to the basic lines and I think you'll find you'll brush away the years.

Here, from Charles Nicholas, owner of the Charles Nicholas Hair Salon in New York City, who has made his international reputation on the basis of his unique ability to solve some of the most challenging styling problems, are some do's and some never-do's for hairstyles guaranteed to make you look years younger.

To Draw Attention Away from Laugh Lines

• A smart choice is a style that pulls hair up to the top of the head and so offsets the lines that pull the face down visually. (Just don't pull hair up too tightly or the look will be too severe.) To do: Put four or five rollers on top of your head—these will help create soft waves that move back away from your face. With rollers still in, collect the hair on the sides and secure with hairpins. Then remove the rollers and brush hair softly back; spread to overlap the sides.

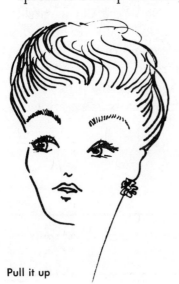

Pull it up

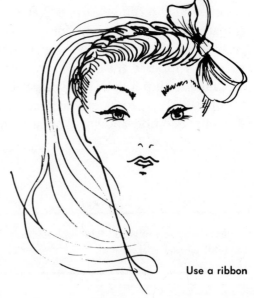

Use a ribbon

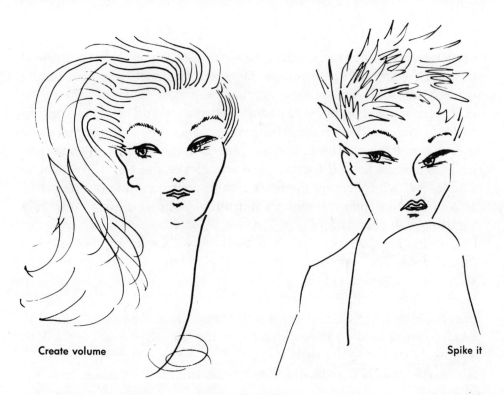

Create volume   Spike it

To color: If the back of your hair is darker than the front, you should add some highlights at the neckline.

· Another good way to hide laugh lines: a style held securely off the face with, say, a twisted scarf or ribbon "anchored" with pincurls fastened with hairpins (easier to conceal than bobby pins). To style: Place one pincurl behind each ear near the hairline; slide the ribbon under these anchors.

To color: Highlights near the hairline and on the crown are great youtheners.

· Use mousse around the hairline for extra hold. When hair is dry, put in a few electric rollers on the full side of the part (to create even more volume), each with a lot of hair on them (so you get fullness, not curl). Leave in for five minutes, remove and finger comb into place.

· Spike it!—and you'll create strong lines in your hair that deemphasize and youthen the real ones on your face. Simply use mousse on your scalp to make hair stand straight up. You might even back-comb the crown for height.

To Erase Forehead Furrows

• Try a one-length blunt cut with a half-bang, and a part over the highest point of the arch of one eyebrow. Mousse or hairspray will provide the control you need to keep the side going away from the face in place.

• Hair is layered with a split wispy bang divided a little off center to concentrate attention on the eyes (a full bang will enhance lines as it conspicuously tries to cover them). The hair at the nape is feathered, too, to soften the neck; sideburns are left long to hide wrinkles at the ear. The styling is simple: Put two rollers on the fuller side of your part, one on the other. Leave in for ten minutes; remove and run your brush through, carefully adjusting with your fingers.

  To color: Highlights on the top of the head will create an all-over taller, thinner look. For very long, thin faces, the addition of highlights on the side, too, will create width.

• Go for a layered cut, shorter on the sides, that falls forward to frame the face, hide lines. Use a little hairspray to keep hair on the sides close to the head, forward on the forehead. To adjust the hair, slide four fingers onto your scalp and bring the roots forward.

  Tip: If your hair is straight and fine, a perm on the front and crown will add volume.

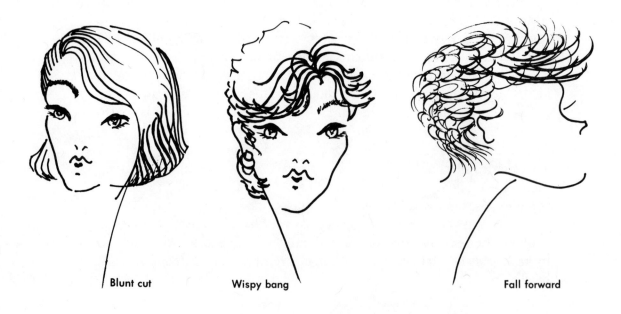

Blunt cut   Wispy bang   Fall forward

To Hide Eye Lines

• A hairstyle that rises at the temples following the upward slant of the cheek-bone creates an optical illusion that almost erases eye lines. Use rollers on the top to create fullness, but set the sides and back with pincurls for tighter, curlier waves.

    To color: Focus coloring on the temples and make it two to three shades lighter than on the rest of the head.

To Uplift a Sagging Chin

• This cut, inspired by Linda Evans's, is designed to draw attention to cheek-bones and detract from the chin. Soft bangs feathered in the center and lifted away from the face on the sides add width (not height); sides are long enough to wrap around the sides of the neck to conceal a sagging jowl. Tip: A good way to control the sides and help them stand away from the face is to hold hair out and spray for twenty seconds; keep holding until it dries and finger comb into place.

    To color: The bangs and crown can go a little lighter; do not highlight near the part (to avoid a dark shadow).

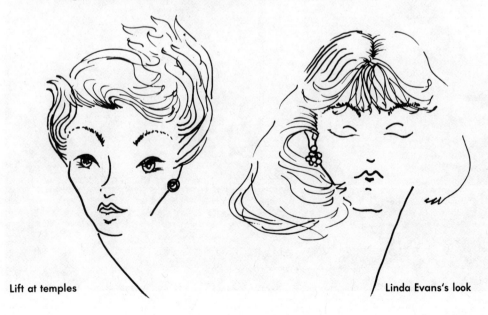

Lift at temples

Linda Evans's look

More ways to conceal a double chin:

· A chin-length bob with a partial perm on the ends will work wonders.
· So will a shorter-than-chin-length cut, side parted with a wave that falls over the forehead.
· In general, layers are a better bet than a blunt cut.

Another uplifting, de-aging style from Lee Bledsoe, owner of Mister Lee Hair Stylist in San Francisco:

First step—color. Streaks were put on the crown to brighten the face. Next, the cut. The top was tapered, shaped slightly shorter over the ears, leaving the back long. Finally, styling. Brushed back and away from the face, this style draws attention to the upper part of the face, provides an instant "lift." Side part contributes an all-over softness.

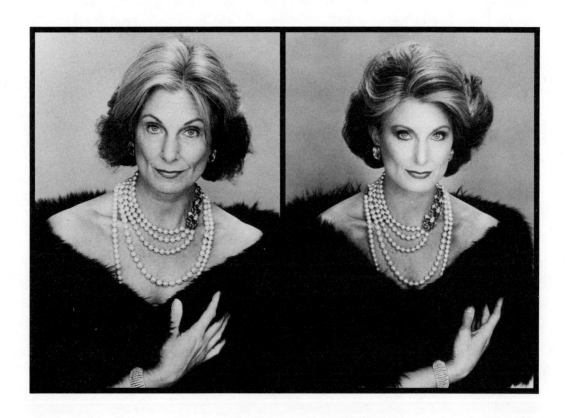

STYLES TO AVOID

- Anything dated, e.g., too-curly or too-bouffant styles; teasing.
- Anything fussy.
- Anything severe.
- Too much hair on the face—it'll look like you're trying to hide something!
- Too-long hair.
- Definite bangs.
- Hair accessories that look too young (like barrettes, clips). They call attention to wrinkles because of their inappropriateness.

SIX

THE ANTIWRINKLE

VITAMIN AND

MINERAL PLAN

I'm not going to give you a beautiful-skin diet plan in the traditional sense—I won't tell you what and how much to eat for breakfast, lunch and dinner to promote younger-looking skin. This is because if you're anything like Catherine and me, your eating patterns are pretty well set . . . for good. You know what's fattening, what's not; what's healthful, what's not; what constitutes a balanced diet and what doesn't—and whether you eat accordingly or not. Some things about your diet are good, some aren't.

What I am going to do is give you the vitamin-and-mineral plan Catherine and I stick to religiously. We think—and many nutritionists have corroborated this—that vitamins and minerals taken in supplementary form with a relatively well balanced diet provide a better and more reliable antiwrinkle diet than any traditional diet plan. The reason: The supplements are specifically antiwrinkle agents in concentrated form. The following five skin-saving vitamins and two minerals are what you need for healthy, youthful skin. Nevertheless, be sure to take them with other vitamins and minerals, too.

Do not just load up on these supplements! It's very important that you consult your doctor and/or nutritionist; he or she will consider your life-style, metabolism, age, stress level and state of health (be sure to indicate whether you're taking any medications, because they might react with or counteract the vitamins and minerals)—and prescribe a balanced vitamin-and-mineral plan specifically for you.

Choosing a Nutritionist
These days everyone is an expert on nutrition and diet. Whom can you rely on for competent professional advice? I asked Meredith Hoblock, a New York City nutritionist and registered dietician.

Your best bet: a registered dietician (R.D.). He or she is a professionally trained nutritionist who has met the educational and professional standards set by the American Dietetic Association. (More and more physicians, usually internists, are specializing in nutrition, too.) An R.D. must have a degree in nutrition or a related science, must have completed an approved dietetic internship or the equivalent, must have passed a national examination and maintained a required number of continuing education hours.

Once you choose a nutritionist, consider him or her part of your regular health care routine. Visits should be ongoing, just like yearly medical check-ups. After all, as your body changes, it only makes sense that your nutritional needs also change.

The key word as far as a vitamin and mineral plan goes is *balanced*. Vitamins and minerals work together to promote health: Overloading on one may diminish another; underproviding one may create a heightened need for another. For example: Since vitamin E assists vitamin A in maintaining the integrity of the body's millions of cells, you have to be careful not to upset this relationship by overdosing on vitamin E, which will create an increased need in the body for more vitamin A.

Once again: For optimal health, vitamins and minerals must be provided in balanced amounts.

SKIN-NOURISHING VITAMINS AND MINERALS
(in order of importance)

vitamin A
vitamin C
vitamin E
vitamin D
B complex
selenium
zinc

Why this particular list? Two reasons: (1) because it contains the *antiaging antioxidants vitamins E and C and the mineral selenium*. Antiaging antioxidants fight "*free radicals*"—highly unstable molecules that, under certain situations in the presence of oxygen, cause cell membrane destruction, a process called cross-linking. Commonly, free radicals attack collagen, the skin's basic support structure. The vitamins E and C and the mineral selenium are natural antioxidants that actually protect the body against collagen breakdown. The mineral zinc, too—though not an antioxidant—is vital for proper collagen synthesis. And (2) because the vitamins A, D, E and B complex generally promote healthy, young-looking skin by improving cell growth, respiration and metabolism.

> **Factors that exacerbate the combining of free radicals with oxygen—and cross-linking—include: exposure to the sun, smoking, and excess consumption of alcohol and coffee.**

SKIN-SAVING VITAMINS AND MINERALS

Coming up is a chart that details how each vitamin and mineral affects the skin, how much you should take . . . and I snuck in food sources, too, so you can see what you should be eating (even if you aren't) and what you shouldn't be eating (even if you are) to get enough of the skin-saving vitamins and minerals into your diet.

Skin-Saving Vitamins and Minerals (in order of importance)	Benefits to the Skin	Daily Dosages/ Recommendations	Food Sources
Vitamin A	Helps keep skin healthy and young-looking by stimulating collagen formation in the dermis; regulating the function of the sebaceous glands, thus assuring well-hydrated skin; protecting against infection; acting as an antioxidant.	• Do not take a vitamin A supplement; instead focus on securing vitamin A from food sources and/or 200 RE (retinol equivalents) of beta carotene, a precursor of vitamin A. Vitamin A is fat soluble and stored by the body; too much can cause toxicity, with side effects including dry skin, headaches, painful swelling of joints.	Green and yellow vegetables (especially carrots, squash, pumpkin); fruits; egg yolks; fortified milk; yogurt; liver.
Vitamin C (Ascorbic Acid)	Natural antioxidant, thus effecting (and maintaining) healthy collagen—and unwrinkled unsaggy skin; ensures the health of capillaries that supply skin with nutrient-rich blood; prevents broken capillaries; plays important role in cellular respiration; like B complex, an antistress vitamin.	• Take 250–500 mg. a day. For every cigarette smoked, add 25 mg. • Avoid chewable varieties because ascorbic acid breaks down tooth enamel • Take supplements with a whole glass of water • Preferably divide dosages in two—one in the morning, one in evening • Vitamin C is highly volatile, is easily destroyed by heat and oxygen and is only stored in the body in very small amounts, so it's absolutely necessary to ingest it on a daily basis • Some people with kidney and bladder problems can develop stones from excess vitamin C supplementation.	Citrus fruits; cantaloupe; berries; watermelon; papaya; green and yellow vegetables (especially broccoli and potatoes).

Skin-Saving Vitamins and Minerals (in order of importance)	Benefits to the Skin	Daily Dosages/ Recommendations	Food Sources
Vitamin E	In conjunction with vitamins A and C, helps retard the aging process by combatting cell and collagen breakdown; protects cells from genetic damage; rebuilds tissues (and builds capillary walls); stimulates cell metabolism, respiration and growth; aids circulation; and protects cell membranes.	• Take 8 mg. a day. Since vitamin E is water soluble and retained by the body, the daily need should not be exceeded (for anyone with high blood pressure or an overactive thyroid, anything in excess of 8 mg. a day could be dangerous) • Exception: You may need more vitamin E if you're in situations that utilize it—if you're in the sun or if you smoke.	Wheat germ; seeds; green leafy vegetables; polyunsaturated oils (corn, safflower, sunflower); whole unrefined grains; eggs; fish.
Vitamin D	Improves skin respiration.	• Take 5 mg. a day • Vitamin D is fat soluble and stored in the body • Do not overdose or you may experience nausea, weakness, kidney stones.	Tuna; milk; salmon; egg yolks; yogurt.
B complex, including: B_1 (thiamin); B_2 (riboflavin); B_3 (niacin); B_6 (pyridoxine); folacin; pantothenic acid; biotin; B_{12} (cobalamin). Note: Complete B complex must be taken and is most effective with vitamins C and E, calcium and phosphorous.	Helps keep skin healthy by improving cellular metabolism, red blood cell formation and cell respiration; controls excessive oiliness and age spots; an antistress vitamin.	• Take a B complex daily that contains 1.1 mg. B_1; 1.1–1.4 mg. B_2; 12–14 mg. B_3; 2 mcg. B_6; 400 mcg. folacin; 10 mg. pantothenic acid; 300 mcg. biotin; 3 mcg. B_{12} • Megadoses can cause flushing and/or itchiness.	Green and yellow vegetables; whole grains; brewer's yeast; yogurt; milk; eggs.
Selenium	Aids vitamins C and E as antioxidants; also involved in cellular respiration and maintenance of red blood cells.	• Take 2 mg. a day.	Eggs; garlic; onion; brewer's yeast; seafood; legumes; whole grains.

Skin-Saving Vitamins and Minerals (in order of importance)	Benefits to the Skin	Daily Dosages/ Recommendations	Food Sources
Zinc	Vital for collagen synthesis, cell growth, oxygen transport and prevention of stretch marks; may also restore natural color to prematurely gray hair.	• Take 15 mg. a day. Too much can lead to iron loss.	Chicken; fish; meat; milk; egg yolks; brewer's yeast; whole grains.

THE IDEAL SKIN-NOURISHING MEAL

I asked Meredith Hoblock to detail the ideal skin-nourishing meal. Her objective was to add moisture to the diet, which keeps skin looking smooth and less lined; to minimize sodium, which contributes to puffiness and bloating; to introduce new foods, textures; to provide foods high in fiber, thereby controlling constipation, which shows up as stress (and lines!) on the skin.

Here it is, complete with recipes and her explanations of why it's good for your skin.

Appetizer: Curried Carrot Soup*
             Whole wheat sesame bread sticks
Entrée: Lotte (monkfish) Florentine*
                and
             Crispy Kasha*
Salad: Confetti Salad* with Lemon-Tofu-Dill Dressing*
Dessert: Fresh Papaya Half with Strawberries and Raspberry Sauce*
             Apricot-Crunch Bar*
Beverage: Sparkling water with lemon or lime wedge
                or
             White wine spritzer

*Recipes follow on pages 138–40.

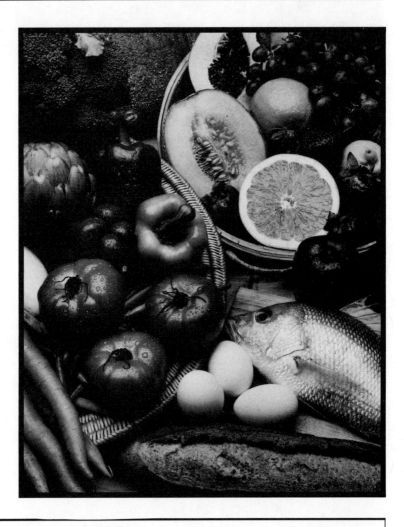

It's an out-and-out myth that if you eat a lot of protein you'll have healthy skin, strong nails and big muscles. You do need the amino acids in proteins (especially the eight essential amino acids your body can't manufacture) for proper growth, repair and maintenance of body tissue . . . but you get ample amounts from less than 50 grams of protein (or 10–15 percent of your total caloric intake). More than that and you have a negative mineral balance and you start losing precious minerals in your body, as well as vital body fluid. Best protein sources are complex carbohydrates—whole grains, mixed seeds and nuts, fruits and vegetables, very lean meats and legumes.

Food/Fluid	Explanation for Inclusion in Ideal Skin-Nourishing Meal
Appetizer: Curried Carrot Soup	Provides fluid, vitamin A, protein, calcium, some B vitamins. Also low in fat and salt. Soup fills you up on relatively few calories; this one is very pretty, too.
Whole wheat sesame bread sticks	Provides fiber, B vitamins, essential oil, carbohydrates. Also low in fat and salt. Adds crunch.
Entrée: Lotte Florentine	Fish cooked in polyunsaturated oil (provides essential oil), herbs and white wine (wine cooks off so no calories, but leaves flavor). Poaching and baking in sauce keep fish moist. Fish provides essential oil, protein, some iron. Also low in fat. Spinach provides fluid, vitamin A, vitamin B; color, flavor; low in salt.
Crispy Kasha	Provides introduction to new grain, vitamins A and B, carbohydrates, protein, calcium; texture, fiber, crunch; low in fat and salt.
Salad: Confetti Salad	Provides fluid, vitamin A, vitamin C, carbohydrates, protein, calcium, essential oil; texture, fiber, crunch, color; low in fact and salt.
Dessert: Fresh Papaya Half with Strawberries and Raspberry Sauce	Provides fluid, vitamin A, vitamin C, carbohydrates, essential oil; texture, fiber, color, sweet taste; low in fat.
Apricot-Crunch Bar	Provides vitamins A and B, carbohydrates, protein, essential oil; texture, fiber, crunch, color, sweet taste.
Beverage: Sparkling water with lemon or lime wedge or	Provides fluid, no calories.
White wine spritzer	Provides fluid, complements meal (fish); low in fat; calms nerves.

CURRIED CARROT SOUP

1 medium yellow onion
2 tablespoons corn, safflower or
   olive oil
4 cups chicken or vegetable broth
1 pound finely chopped carrots

1 teaspoon curry powder
½ cup low-fat yogurt
1 teaspoon grated lemon rind

Sauté onion in oil until golden. Add broth and heat to boiling. Stir in finely chopped carrots and simmer for 20 minutes. In a blender or food processor puree broth mixture, half at a time. (At this point you may cover and refrigerate for up to two days.)

To serve, return soup to pan; add curry and yogurt and bring to a simmer—do not boil—stirring occasionally.

Garnish with grated lemon rind.

Makes 5 cups (4–6 servings).

CRISPY KASHA (OR OTHER GRAIN)

1 medium onion, chopped
1 clove garlic, minced
¼ pound mushrooms, chopped
2 tablespoons minced fresh
   coriander leaves
1 tablespoon safflower or
   sunflower oil
⅔ cup rice (brown, preferably)

⅓ cup kasha (or other grain)
1 cup cubed raw zucchini
½ cup sunflower seeds
2½ cups vegetable broth or 1 cup
   chicken broth plus ½ cup white
   wine plus 1 cup water

Sauté onion, garlic, mushrooms and coriander in oil until golden; add brown rice and kasha. Stir until lightly toasted. Add zucchini, sunflower seeds and vegetable broth. Cover and simmer for about 20 minutes.

Makes 4 servings.

LOTTE FLORENTINE

2 pounds lotte (monkfish) fillets
2 1/2 cups water
1/2 cup dry white wine
1 leek, shredded (reserve half for sauce)
1 pound spinach leaves, washed well, stems removed
1 medium onion, chopped fine
2 tablespoons olive oil

1/2 cup low-fat yogurt
3 tablespoons cooking sherry
Dash cayenne pepper
1/4 cup dry whole wheat bread crumbs
1 tablespoon wheat germ
1 tablespoon Parmesan cheese

Poach fish in barely simmering water, wine and 1/2 of shredded leek for 25 minutes; remove from heat and drain, reserving cooking fluid. Cut fish into bite-size pieces and place in a lightly oiled casserole on top of fresh spinach leaves.

Preheat oven to 350° F. Sauté remaining leek and onion in oil until translucent. Add reserved fish fluid to sautéed leek—onion mixture and bring to a boil. Reduce to a simmer. Slowly stir in yogurt, cooking sherry and cayenne. Pour over fish in casserole. Mix bread crumbs, wheat germ and cheese, and scatter on top of fish. Put casserole in oven and bake until sauce bubbles and crumbs are brown.

Makes 4 servings.

CONFETTI SALAD

1/2 head red leaf lettuce
1/2 bunch watercress, stems attached
1 green pepper

1/2 head red cabbage
Lemon-Tofu-Dill Dressing (recipe follows)

Wash, dry and break red leaf lettuce and watercress into bite-size pieces. Thinly slice green pepper and shred red cabbage. Toss all together and top with Lemon-Tofu-Dill Dressing.

Makes 4 servings.

LEMON-TOFU-DILL DRESSING

2½ ounces tofu
2 tablespoons lemon juice
1 tablespoon olive oil

½ clove garlic, mashed
2 tablespoons water
1 tablespoon fresh dill

Cream all ingredients in a blender or food processor. Add water to reduce thickness if necessary.

RASPBERRY SAUCE (FOR FRESH PAPAYA HALF WITH STRAWBERRIES)

½ cup orange juice
1 cup water
½ pint fresh raspberries, pureed

1 teaspoon grated lemon rind
½ teaspoon cassis or kirsch

Heat orange juice and water to a boil. Stir in pureed berries and lemon rind. Cook for 15 minutes over low flame. Add cassis and stir. Remove from heat and allow sauce to cool to room temperature.
Makes 4 servings.
To assemble dessert: Cut papaya in half lengthwise. Scoop out seeds and discard. Fill cavity with strawberries (tops removed). Spoon raspberry sauce over strawberries.

APRICOT-CRUNCH BARS

2 whole medium eggs
1 egg white
⅔ cup raspberry jam
⅓ cup unsweetened applesauce
⅔ cup whole wheat flour
¼ cup toasted wheat germ

½ cup regular oatmeal
1 teaspoon safflower oil
1 teaspoon vanilla
½ cup coarsely chopped almonds
2 cups chopped dried apricots

Preheat oven to 325° F. Beat eggs until light and fluffy. Add jam and applesauce. Blend well. Stir in flour, wheat germ and oatmeal gradually until well blended. Add oil and vanilla. Stir in almonds and apricots. Pour batter into lightly oiled and floured 9 by 13-inch pan. Bake for about 25 minutes. When cool, cut into bars.
Makes 42 2½ by 1-inch bars.

The truth about RDAs

Nutrition is a very young science (only about 25 years old), and in order to determine what human beings need in terms of specific nutrients, extensive studies on a wide variety of people would have to be done, Meredith Hoblock told me. However, since using humans for experiments is illegal, we have to rely on animal studies, which are only so transferrable to the human system as requirements and utilization of nutrients go.

So the bottom line on RDAs (Recommended Daily Allowances) is that while some may be adequate, many aren't. In general, they're low because they're based on a perfectly balanced diet, and if you aren't eating one—who is?— they're off. But they're all we have . . . and they're a good place for nutritionists to start: Go to one—don't have the man or woman behind the health food counter prescribe what you should and shouldn't be taking.

Consider Drinking Your Vitamins

Two great suppliers of hard-to-get nutrients: parsley (just ½ cup contains all the vitamins A, B, C you need a day); and carrots (rich in vitamins B, C, D and E—four carrots a day will keep your skin looking the way you like it!).

How to increase your intake: Try drinking a glass of carrot juice with a squeeze of lemon juice every morning for four to six weeks and I guarantee you'll see a change in your complexion. Get into the habit, too, of mixing parsley into salads and into yogurt for a super potato topper, substituting it for basil in pesto or stirring it into a tomato or primavera sauce.

Here, also from Meredith Hoblock, is one of the best beauty drinks I know:

SKIN-SAVING STRAWBERRY-APRICOT SHAKE

½ cup fresh strawberries (high in
  vitamin C)
1 fresh apricot, pitted (high in
  vitamin A)
1 tablespoon wheat germ (high in
  vitamin E)

¼ cup vanilla yogurt (high in
  protein, vitamins B_2, B_{12})

Blend all ingredients.
Makes 1 serving.

Brewer's yeast is one of the most beauty boosting foods around, but many brands are so tasteless they make consuming brewer's yeast a real chore. Catherine and I make a drink with it: Take ¼ teaspoon yeast and mix it into 6 ounces of low-sodium V-8 or unsweetened grapefruit juice. It's not bad. (Yeast should be taken slowly at first or it may create gas and bloat; so after a week increase the yeast to ½ teaspoon and continue to increase by ½ teaspoon every day until you're taking 3 tablespoons a day.) A note of interest: Almost twenty years ago Benjamin S. Frank, M.D., was prescribing doses of RNA (usually taken from yeast) in combination with other vitamins and minerals to reverse the symptoms of aging. At the time many doctors found this laughable. No more, though!

Beauty Fats

A lot is being said these days about fats. Two issues are important here—the total amount of fat you consume daily and the type of fat.

Dietary fat has been linked to cancers of the breast and colon as well as to heart disease. For optimal health, no more than 30 percent of your daily calories should come from fat. Of this, 20 percent should come from poly- and monounsaturated fats—essential fatty acids (EFAs) that are necessary for young-looking skin. They provide the chemical building blocks of cell membranes and intercellular cement; ensure the exchange of oxygen and nutrients from the blood to the skin cells; help skin retain moisture; and strengthen the immune system (important in preventing premature signs of aging).

Foods containings EFAs are vegetable oils like safflower, soy, corn and olive oils; wheat germ; and oily fish such as mackerel. In addition to including these foods in your diet, it's important that (1) your diet include an adequate supply of vitamins C, B_6 and niacin and the minerals zinc and magnesium— the nutrients that convert essential fats into their biologically active forms; and (2) your diet should be as free as possible of saturated fats, which keep EFAs from being assimilated by the body. While unsaturated fats are usually in the form of liquid vegetable oils, saturated fats are found in solid animal fats (meat and dairy products), in highly processed fats such as margarine and vegetable shortening and in foods containing them. These foods have undergone "hydrogenation," which turns unsaturated oils to a more solid (saturated form) of fat.

Note: As with everything, there are exceptions to the rules. Not all unsaturates are good for you. How to tell which are, which aren't: It depends on how much linoleic acid is present. The higher the linoleic content, the greater the degree of polyunsaturation and the better it'll be for your skin. Some safflower oils, for example, are 75 percent linoleic acid, while others (high oleic safflower oil) are only 14 percent linoleic. (FYI: Butter, a bad saturated fat, is 2 percent linoleic acid.) Reading labels should help clue you in to the percentage of linoleic acid contained in the product; when the information is not available, stay away from products with palm and coconut oils.

Carl C. Pfeiffer, M.D., Ph.D., of the Princeton Brain Bio Center, advocates Max EPA (which is available at most health food stores) to improve dry skin from the inside out. It's a concentrate of fish oils containing elcosapentaenoic acid (EPA). Take Max EPA with British Evening Primrose Oil, two 10-gram capsules of each every day. His new research shows that molybdenum and magnesium may have a profound effect on preventing skin from aging as well. He suggests taking 500 micrograms of molybdenum once a day, and magnesium in the form of Milk of Magnesia tablets three times a day.

WRINKLE-REVERSING ENZYMES

Up until very recently it's been thought that skin damage was irreversible. No more! *Damaged skin can be restored!*

Here's why: Half your collagen supply is replaced every five to seven years with a new supply that's as strong (and young-looking) as a baby's, so if you could step up that replacement process, you could repair damaged skin.

Two enzymes, bromelain and papain, found in fresh pineapple and papaya, do just that—they actually dissolve the old damaged collagen and incite the body to produce new, healthy collagen fibers in skin-supportive, orderly rows.

You can eat the fruits raw (the riper they are, the higher their concentration of enzymes). Just don't go overboard: If your mouth becomes sore and tender, you've eaten too much . . . and don't eat either if you have an ulcer (they speed the rate at which protein is digested, slowing healing). You can also apply them topically for the same effect. After smoothing on a moisturizer, which acts as a "carrier" for the enzymes, rub skin with a slice or two of fresh pineapple or mashed papaya for one minute; cleanse with regular cleanser.

Or try this drink from Sonoma Mission Inn and Spa:

PAPAYA-PINEAPPLE SLUSH

¼ ripe medium papaya, seeded and skinned
½ cup fresh ripe pineapple, cubed
1 tablespoon fresh lemon juice

1 teaspoon honey, if desired
Crushed ice

Blend all ingredients except ice until smooth. Add crushed ice until mixture attains slush consistency.
Makes 2 servings.

WATER—THE BEST MOISTURIZER OF ALL

Besides hydrating skin cells, another water bonus is that it cleans the cells, actually flushing out your system through perspiration—it is, in fact, a kind of diuretic . . . the only "good" diuretic. When waste products build up, they impede microcirculation to the skin (as opposed to macrocirculation to the rest of the organs), decreasing the amount of nutrients carried to the cells as well as reducing waste eliminated from the cells. The result is tissue sludge that further slows cellular activity.

Many women feel that if they retain fluids they should stay away from water—no! They should stay away from salt!

How much water is enough water? Six to eight glasses of tap water, seltzer or low-sodium mineral water or herbal tea spaced throughout a day; more if you can manage it. In other words: No amount of water is too much. Coffee, nonherbal teas, soft drinks and/or alcoholic beverages are not substitutes for water because they all contain caffeine, which is a diuretic and causes you to lose fluid.

I drink hot water with lemon slices. I remember my grandmother drinking this every morning and every night before bed: She swore by its cleansing effects.

Catherine says a lot of models and actresses she interviewed when she was at *Bazaar* told her they drink hot lemon water by the gallon.

What to do if you can't drink past your thirst-quench quota? Water down all your liquids (from your morning juice to wine with dinner) with half seltzer—you'll slash calories in addition to ensuring proper skin cell hydration. Also increase your intake of mostly vitamin-A and -C rich fruits and vegetables that themselves contain high percentages of water. Some numbers will be found in the chart on the following page.

Fruits (% water)	Vegetables (% water)
cantaloupe—91%	tomatoes—93%
strawberries—90%	asparagus—92%
papaya—89%	green beans—92%
peaches—89%	alfalfa sprouts—91%
apricots—85%	carrots—88%
raspberries—84%	artichokes—87%
kiwi—83%	corn—74%
pears—83%	
Also good: whole milk—80%	

In winter many people, because they're not hot and don't sweat, drink less water than usual. Very bad! This is a time when you should drink lots of water, more even than what's prescribed as "normal," to keep skin hydrated from the inside out. Cold dry winter air and wind plus steam heat are serious moisture robbers.

THREE-DAY SKIN-IMPROVING MINIFAST

Because water is the ultimate cleanser for your body (and your skin), I am going to give you a three-day water-based skin purge, which Catherine and I asked Meredith Hoblock to design for us. I don't recommend fasts and feel regimented diets are an imposition (and unnecessary if you have a basic understanding of nutrition), but I do feel that an occasional 500-calorie-a-day fast like this after a few "bad" days is great for getting you back on track. On pages 148–49, you'll find the Hoblock minifast Catherine and I use after the holidays and after vacations. (If you need a more intense purge to detoxify your skin after more than just a few days of too much fat and protein, refined carbohydrates and alcohol, try a ten-day to two-week diet that's low in fat and protein; avoid sugar, white flour and alcohol.) *Do not do the three-day purge for any longer than three days!*

What the diet will do for you and your skin:

- Detoxify the body of toxins, drugs, artificial sweeteners, caffeine, sodium, chemical additives.
- Introduce balanced skin-nourishing nutrients.
- Increase moisture content of body.
- Give the body a rest from an abusive eating regimen, e.g., unbalanced/haphazard habits.
- Taper off caffeine dependence.

During the three days, intense exercise should be kept to a minimum, but walking is encouraged as much as possible.

Don't be surprised if you're headachy, even nauseous at the beginning of your fast—this is just a good indication that your body is detoxifying. You may even feel slightly dizzy as your circulation and heart rate slow (your brain isn't getting as much blood as it's used to). On the other hand, you may feel your heart beating too fast. Simply rest, and if symptoms persist, have a glass of juice. Once again, do not do the Three-Day Skin-Improving Minifast for any longer than three days, and, of course, it should go without saying: no toxins (that is, no smoking, drinking and/or drugs). And note, too, that nobody with kidney disease, bleeding ulcers or diabetes should fast.

How to Lose Weight, Not Your Looks
A prominent nutritionist in Los Angeles, Hermien Lee, has all her overweight patients eat a mix of at least three varieties of raw or lightly steamed vegetables daily when dieting. The vitamins and minerals in the vegetables help save the skin during weight loss.

500-Calorie Three-Day Menu Plan for Skin-Improving Minifast			
Meal	Day 1	Day 2	Day 3
Breakfast	Fruit drink: In a blender, mix 4 ounces grapefruit juice (40 cals.), 1 tablespoon skim milk powder (30 cals.), ½ mango or 1 medium peach (20 cals.), 4 oz. cold water	1 thin slice whole wheatberry toast (21 cals.) topped with ½ cup unsweetened applesauce sprinkled with cinnamon (53 cals.)	½ cup cooked oatmeal (52 cals.) ¼ cup raspberries (15 cals.) 2 tablespoons skim milk (10 cals.) ½ teaspoon brown sugar (9 cals.)
Calories	90 cals.	74 cals.	86 cals.
Mid-morning	1 cup watermelon balls (50 cals.) mixed with ½ cup honeydew balls (30 cals.)	Tomato-Vegetable Juice: In a blender, mix 6 ounces tomato juice (30 cals.), 2 ounces cold water, ¼ cup grated zucchini and cucumber (25 cals.)	½ papaya (40 cals.) filled with ¼–½ cup berries in season (blueberries—40 cals.)
Calories	80 cals.	55 cals.	80 cals.
Lunch	½ medium tomato (25 cals.) stuffed with mixture of 2 tablespoons cooked brown rice (17 cals.), 1 tablespoon lowfat plain yogurt (10 cals.), 2 teaspoons sunflower seeds (26 cals.), 1 tablespoon cooked lentils (11 cals.), 1 tablespoon grated zucchini (5 cals.)	Carrot Raisin Salad: ½ cup grated large carrots (25 cals.) mixed with 2 tablespoons raisins (40 cals.) and 1 tablespoon lowfat plain yogurt (10 cals.), stuffed into 1 small sesame whole wheat pita (60 cals.)	Spinach Soup: ½ cup cooked spinach (25 cals.) pureed with 1 tablespoon plain yogurt (10 cals.), 2 ounces water, dash nutmeg, topped with ½ cooked egg, sliced (37 cals.) and 1 whole wheat sesame breadstick (25 cals.)
Calories	94 cals.	135 cals.	97 cals.

500-Calorie Three-Day Menu Plan for Skin-Improving Minifast			
Meal	Day 1	Day 2	Day 3
Mid-afternoon	Fruit Juice Cocktail: Mix together 2 ounces apricot nectar (29 cals.), 4 ounces cold water, 3 ounces orange juice (30 cals.)	¼ cantaloupe (40 cals.), cubed and tossed with 8 red grapes (26 cals.)	In a bowl, mix together 4 dried apricot halves (30 cals.) with 4 raw almonds, oven toasted (25 cals.)
Calories	59 cals.	66 cals.	55 cals.
Dinner	1 cup steamed broccoli, pea pods, carrots (50 cals.) 1 ounce tofu, mashed (22 cals.) with ½ teaspoon Italian dressing (herbs, lemon and sunflower oil) (15 cals.)	½ cup cooked spaghetti squash (60 cals.) topped with ¼ cup tomato puree (25 cals.), 2 mushrooms, chopped (10 cals.), 1 teaspoon Parmesan cheese (15 cals.)	Cold Rice Salad: ½ cup cooked brown rice (64 cals.) mixed with ¼ cup green pepper, cubed (12 cals.), ½ ounce chicken, cubed (25 cals.), and ½ teaspoon safflower oil (20 cals.) mashed into 1 tablespoon tofu (11 cals.)
Calories	87 cals.	110 cals.	132 cals.
Before bed	1 fresh apple (90 cals.)	Orange Sparkle: In a blender, mix 4 ounces fresh orange juice (40 cals.), 2 ounces water, 2 slices (¼") kiwi (20 cals.)	Cranberry Juice Spritzer: Mix 3 ounces cranberry juice cocktail (50 cals.) with 3 ounces sparkling water
Calories	90 cals.	60 cals.	50 cals.

SEVEN

THE ANTIWRINKLE

TAN PLAN

I for one love the look of a tan. And let's face it: In this day and age, when being beautiful is in large measure determined by looking healthy and fit, pale just isn't as pretty as tan. But can you tan without completely damaging your skin? The answer: an irrefutable—and resounding—yes.

In fact, one of the best forms of protection from the sun is a light tan!

After talking to dozens of dermatologists, both practicing and researching; plastic surgeons; Ph.D.s (chemists, biologists and physicists); and other skin care experts (particularly aestheticians), I've put together a foolproof, healthy antiwrinkle tan plan. But before I get to it, I want to fill you in on some of the details that determined its final form.

WHAT THE SUN DOES TO THE SKIN

Up until very recently the consensus among the medical profession was that sun damage—that is, the degeneration of the skin's support system of collagen and elastin fibers—was solely the result of UV-B rays, the ultraviolet rays largely responsible for burning. Now, though, it's thought that UV-A rays, which are responsible for tanning, are equally—if not more!—harmful. (The other ultraviolet rays, UV-C, are almost entirely filtered out by the atmosphere.) In fact, 50 percent of UV-A rays are diffused in the epidermis and actually augment the burning effects of UV-B (only 30 percent of UV-B rays are diffused in the epidermis), and recently it has been found that UV-A penetrates the dermis even more deeply than UV-B. So both are responsible for sun damage.

A new ray has been identified and is suspected to cause the same damage to skin as UV light: It is infrared light. Whereas you see UV light, you feel infrared light in the form of heat. It is the "hot" ray (UV is the "cool" ray), and the hotter you get in the sun, the worse the damage to your skin (almost 50 percent of the sun's radiation is infrared). To date, no product has been developed to absorb it. Dr. Kligman told me a whole new generation of sun screens will have to be developed. These new products—sort of sun paints— will have to contain pigments—blue! yellow!—to reflect these rays.

Another new finding, which came as a big surprise to me: The accumulation of normal light—not just direct sunlight absorbed by sunbathing—is very damaging to the skin. In fact, it's thought that upward of 70 percent of the sun damage (from both UV-A and UV-B rays) that you incur over your lifetime is done during everyday activities—walking, driving, even sitting in your sun-drenched living room (when sunlight comes through a window, its intensity can actually double as it bounces off reflective surfaces). This finding is at least in part responsible for cosmetics companies adding sun screens to most of their products. Why take unnecessary risks? It's simple to choose a moisturizer with the built-in protection of a sun screen over one without it. And a lot of makeup, too, is being formulated to absorb both UV-A and UV-B rays before they can penetrate your skin.

The point, then, should be obvious: Protect yourself from the sun. As long as you expose yourself to the sun unprotected—that means being out without an adequate sun screen and being out so long you become greatly over-heated—damage continues. Once you stop, damage stops and repair begins because the skin is always renewing itself, always producing new collagen. Thus you can stop sun damage at *any age!*

Winter Sunburn! Help!

Unfortunately, so much emphasis has been put on the damaging effects of summer sun, we've gotten into the habit of ignoring the effects of winter sun, which can be equally hazardous. Never underestimate the intensity of snow's reflective powers (it's about 90 percent higher when you're in high altitudes, say, skiing, where the air is thin) or the doubly damaging effects of sun on skin dehydrated by low humidity and/or high winds!

So, whenever you're going to be outside in winter—be it skiing, skating or just walking about—follow the tan plan coming up as carefully as you do in summer. In fact, you'd be wise to do so even more diligently in winter. In the first place, the cold may make you forget that sun damage is taking place; combine this with the facts that the thick layer of protective cells your skin builds up over the summer is now gone and that oil production, which speeds up in summer, slows in winter, and you're without any natural barrier against the elements . . . and all that much more susceptible to sun damage.

And: Winter conditions—the combination of sun, wind, dry air and cold temperatures—dry and crack skin, making the lines you already have that much more prominent.

WHAT THE NEW SUN SCREENS CAN DO FOR YOU

Until very recently almost all the available sun screens protected only against UV-B rays, allowing you to be in the sun without burning, sure, but allowing damage, too, because they permit damaging UV-A tanning rays to penetrate. So the bottom line has been that no matter how well you "protected" yourself, you were, indeed, still damaging your skin.

Now, however, there are products that protect against both UV-A and UV-B rays, letting everyone tan without burning . . . and without incurring damage. Since many of the old UV-B–only screens are still on the market, it's important that you learn how to identify these new products. Many are labeled "broad spectrum." Check ingredients, too: Oxybenzone is a UV-A blocker.

In addition to these products, there is a whole new category of pre-sun products you can begin using a few days before exposure to produce extra melanin so that you tan darker, faster, even with a sun screen with an SPF of 15. So for maximum protection here's what I suggest: Use one of these new pre-sun melanin-producing products in conjunction with one of the new "broad spectrum" sun screens. And, after exposure, if you want to prolong your tan, there's yet another new category of sun products called tan maintainers, which, working on the same principle of stimulating melanin production, keep you tanner longer even after sun exposure is over.

I'm sure you know by now what SPF (sun protection factor) refers to, but to refresh: A product's SPF extends the length of time you can stay out in the sun without burning. An SPF of 2 means you can stay out twice as long with the product as without it before you'll burn; an SPF of 15 means 15 times as long.

Smart Sun Screening

I have a confession to make: Even though I was telling *Bazaar* readers never to go outside without a sun screen, I was reluctant to wear one for years. I like having a little color; it makes me look better and feel better. But as I neared forty and saw more and more lines forming, I decided I'd better start taking my own advice. So I started using a sun screen with a high SPF—usually 15—and to my surprise I still got some color.

Sun screens are now available with SPFs that range from 2 to 23 (the higher the SPF, the more UV-B–absorbing PABA it contains). To find out which factor is right for you, check the chart on page 160.

(Note that about 5 percent of the population is allergic to PABA, para-aminobenzoic acid, or one of its chemical derivatives. PABA, in combination with sunlight, can cause red, itchy, blotchy patches on the skin of allergic persons. If you suspect you may be allergic to it, do a patch test: Put a drop of the product on the inside of your arm or on your back. Cover with a bandage for forty-eight hours. If a rash turns up, see your dermatologist and look for a sun screen with alternative ingredients.)

Whichever SPF you choose, consider, too, which formulation is right for your skin type, needs and preferences. *If you have oily skin,* go for a gel. *If you have dry skin,* try a cream-based formula. Either way, my recommendation is to stay away from the oils—they tend to trap body heat and form tiny beads of moisture that act like magnifying glasses to intensify the damaging effects of the sun.

Almost as important as picking the proper SPF and formulation is applying a sun screen properly. If you don't, you could negate all your good intentions. Here, some tips to help you maximize your sun screen's effectiveness:

- *Don't wash or exfoliate immediately before applying sun screen.* You'll remove dead surface skin cells that bind the protective ingredients to your skin and serve as a barrier against burning, too.
- *Plan ahead.* Sun screens should be put on at least 30 minutes (preferably 2 hours) before exposure begins. Never wait until after you're outside to apply it. Chances are you will have been out long enough for a burn to get well underway; plus, you will have started to perspire, which reduces the potency of the screen. Don't forget that while some PABA stays on the surface of the skin, some will penetrate, but it'll take time. Repeated daily use will result in a buildup of PABA in the stratum corneum . . . and added protection.
- *Don't rub the sun screen in!* It should be a film on the surface of your skin, just thick enough to form a protective layer: It must serve as a filter.
- *Apply sun screen twice.* This is a tip from Catherine, who learned the hard way. When she was skiing once, she applied her sun screen but forgot her chin—and paid dearly with a severe burn. A second application will cover the spots the first application missed.
- *Reapply frequently during the day, too.* Catherine reapplies her sun screen every time she goes up the mountain when she's skiing. She's right: Whether you're skiing, playing tennis or golf or just strolling on a pleasant afternoon, you'll probably sweat, which in itself will wash off sun screens (SPFs do not take humidity or perspiration into account), or you may wipe your brow and so wipe away your protection. You must reapply your sun screen . . . and that goes for products labeled water resistant, too. A final note on reapplication: Putting on more sun

---

New sun screens in the works: (1) A simple product that would block not only UV-A and UV-B rays but infrared, too. These products will probably contain pigments, making them bright blue or yellow to reflect the sun. (2) A single-application sun screen (to be applied before bedtime the night before exposure) that would change the composition of the stratum corneum so it would itself block out the sun's damaging rays; benefits would last for 3 to 6 days. (3) A sun screen pill that would prevent sunburning as well as cancer-causing changes in skin composition. (4) Prescription pills containing psoralen, to be taken two days before sun exposure to prevent sunburning.

screen with an SPF of, say, 15 does not increase the length of time you can be in the sun without burning: It simply reinstates the original protection factor.

- Consider eating your sun screen! New research has shown that vitamins C, E and pyridoxine, and beta carotene, the precursor of vitamin A, help you build up natural resistance to the burning effects of the sun.
- *Pay special attention to eyes and lips.* They're the most often forgotten spots. Here, some special tips for screening them from the sun:

EYES

- The skin around your eyes is so thin and delicate that a sun screen alone isn't enough protection. I've found that a sun screen made for lips works wonders on eyes, too, because of its waxy consistency. (Until I discovered this I often avoided screening my eyes because perspiration used to make my regular sun screen run, work it's way into my eyes—and sting.) Plus lip sun screen is portable! Just make sure you use one with an SPF of 15 or higher.
- To keep sun screen from running into your eyes and irritating them, powder over it! Or try one of the new sun screens made specifically for eyes—they're eye-friendly because they're anhydrous (that is, contain no water), will stay put and, what's more, can easily be flushed out of the eye if some does seep in.

  Tip: If you have crow's-feet, don't let them tan at all—the sun won't fill in the lines, and they'll appear whiter than tanned skin around them . . . and they'll look more pronounced than ever.

LIPS

- Lip skin, really exposed mucous membrane, contains little if any melanin. Combine that fact with the fact of saliva on the lips and/or the common habit of frequently licking lips and you intensify the burning effects of the sun on this area. What lips need: a sun screen with an SPF of 15 or above specifically formulated for lips; these formulations have a waxy base that seals in moisture, won't be diluted by saliva. Look for products with jojoba oil, vitamins A and E and aloe.
- Wearing lipstick (not gloss) is a help also (the thicker you put it on, the better). Best color choices (because they contain a lot of sun-blocking pigments): reds, pinks, peaches, corals.

MY WRINKLE-PROOF FOUR-STEP TAN PLAN

1. Do you think that once you're tan you're home free, that no more damage is being done to your skin and that you no longer need protection from the sun?
2. Do you think you are less likely to burn on a breezy, cool day when the sky's hazy than on a very hot, clear, scorcher of a day?
3. Do you think that if you swim mostly underwater, say, if you're snorkeling, you're safe (and hidden) from the sun's burning rays?

One yes and you're all wrong! . . . and a prime candidate for my new healthy tan plan. Here are the reasons the nos won.

1. Just because you have a tan doesn't mean UV damage has stopped. Even tanned skin needs protection: A tan doesn't cover the entire surface of the skin; it's blotchy. And so those spots that aren't tan are susceptible to sun damage.
2. Surprisingly, even though on hazy days only 50 percent of UV radiation reaches the earth compared with 100 percent on clear days, you're probably less likely to burn on a scorcher than on a cooler day: The heat will drive you out of the sun and into a shadier, more comfortable place.
3. Actually, since ultraviolet rays go straight through water, even snorkelers and skindivers are subject to severe burning.

Following is my Tan Plan. Its four steps are so simple and easy to follow, they'll become second nature before you know it. They'll let you tan safely, healthily and beautifully. Remember: Though pale isn't as pretty as a sun-kissed golden glow, neither is the brown, baked look that was so popular years ago.

Step 1. Find your own sun susceptibility.

For years I was under the impression that my Italian heritage— my dark-skinned complexion, dark hair and eyes—exempted me from sunburning and sun damage. I was wrong. True, many of my friends with dark thick skin, dark hair and dark eyes always tanned beautifully and rarely burned, but I burned badly and rarely tanned.

As far as sun susceptibility goes, looks can be deceiving. For example, if you're fair and blond, you may think you're a prime candidate for getting burned to a crisp when, in fact, you may have more melanin than someone who's darkly complected with dark hair.

How to see your burn potential? Your eyes tell all. Generally, light-eyed people have less tolerance to the sun than dark-eyed people. Here's a further breakdown:

You burn easily, tan rarely (absorb about 45 % of the sun's rays) if you have . . .	You burn minimally, tan gradually (absorb about 35% of the sun's rays) if you have . . .	You tan easily, burn rarely (absorb about 20% of the sun's rays) if you have . . .
• blue or green eyes • thin, sensitive, see-through skin • dry (or normal) skin • small pores	• green or brown eyes • medium-thick skin • normal (or combination) skin • medium-size pores	• dark brown or black eyes • thick, durable skin • oily complexion • large pores

Step 2. Determine your own sun sensitivity.

Now that you've determined how susceptible you are to sunburning, it's important to consider how reactive (or photosensitive) your skin is to sunlight—that is, how your skin, in combination with another agent taken internally or applied externally, reacts when it's exposed to the sun. *Note:* In addition to being sensitive to the sun plus another agent, you can be sensitive to the sun itself. This does not mean that you burn but that you burn extremely badly and/or react with a severe allergic reaction.

Say you tan easily and rarely burn. You may not always do so: You could easily—and immediately—become super sun-sensitive and burn to a crisp if you are using a photosensitizing product. Beware of photosensitizers! If you're taking or using any, stay out of the sun and/or switch to medications or products that are not photosensitive. (Topical applications of cortico-steroid can be helpful if a reaction is incurred.)

Here, a list of the most common offenders. Be aware that reactions vary with every individual—in fact, you may not react at all.

You May Be Sun-Sensitive if You Are Using . . .

These potentially phototoxic drugs	These potentially photoallergenic products
· antibiotics of the tetracycline family · antidepressants · antihistamines · birth control pills · Retin-A, a derivative of vitamin A acid · sulfa drugs and sulfa derivatives such as thiazide diuretics and the oral hypoglycemic agents (taken by some diabetics) · sulfonamides (usually prescribed for urinary tract infections)	· antibacterial deodorant soaps containing halogenated salicylanilides · perfumes and colognes with bergamot, sandalwood, lavender and/or citron oils. *Tip:* Never go into the sun with lemon or lime juice on your skin (say, if you've put some on your hair or if you've just squeezed some into a drink)—they can cause terrible burns. · plants such as ragweed, carrots, parsnips, parsley, fennel and figs (also celery, dill and mustard) · skin-bleaching creams (for brown spots or other kinds of hyperpigmentation) · tar-based antiseptic creams · tar-based detergents · tar-based shampoos

Step 3. Calculate the sun's intensity.

If you spend your summers in the northern parts of the United States—in Cape Cod, for example, or on the shores of the Great Lakes or in the Pacific Northwest—you may, indeed, tan beautifully. But what happens if you head south or high up into the mountains? What happens if you go to the Caribbean or Mexico in the dead of winter? Use the same protection you usually use and you may (literally) fry. Here's how to tell when sun is most damaging.

	Sun is most damaging . . .
Time of day	Between 11 A.M. and 3 P.M. When the sun is directly overhead, the distance the rays must travel to reach you is shorter (and, therefore, more damaging) than when it's "higher" in the sky.
Time of year	Late spring/early–mid summer. The earth is closest to the sun around June 21, the first day of summer.
Altitude	In high altitudes. The air is less dense than at sea level, plus there's no haze and pollution to filter out burning rays.
Latitude	The closer you are to the equator. Radiation is $1\frac{1}{2}$ times greater, for example, in the southern United States than in the northern United States.
Humidity	In dry air, which is transparent, letting the sun's rays penetrate easily. That's why the sun is so intense in the dry desert or in high mountains.

The Weekend Tan
What to do if you're getting your tan from weekend to weekend? The first and second weekends out, develop a base tan (see the chart, p. 160) with the sun screen prescribed for your skin's sun susceptibility. If you're sun sensitive, stay with your sun block. If you burn easily, tan rarely, stick with your base-tan SPF through the third weekend until the fourth weekend, when you can drop to an SPF 10. If you burn minimally, tan gradually or tan easily, burn rarely, you can go to SPF 8 on the third weekend. Continue with lower SPFs.

Step 4. Follow our Tan Plan. Turn the page . . .

If you . . .

	Are sun sensitive	Burn easily, tan rarely	Burn minimally, tan gradually	Tan easily, burn rarely
Without a proper sun screen on day 1, you'll burn in this amount of time*	10–15 minutes	15 minutes	20 minutes	25 minutes
Days 1–3 (to develop a base)	• Wear a total block or a product with SPF 15–23. • If you're allergic to the sun itself (as opposed to being sensitive to the sun plus another agent—see p. 158), be sure you're using a broad spectrum sun screen and confine sunning to before noon and after 3 P.M.	• Use a sun screen with SPF 15. • Time of exposure: up to 3 hours 45 minutes before you begin to burn.	• Use a sun screen with SPF 10. • Time of exposure: up to 3 hours 30 minutes before you begin to burn.	• Use a sun screen with SPF 8. • Time of exposure: up to 3 hours 20 minutes before you begin to burn.
After 3 days (to maintain your base)	• Same as above.	• SPF 8.	• SPF 8.	• SPF 6.
After 3 days (to get and maintain a *darker* color than the base color)	• Same as above.	• SPF 6.	• SPF 6.	• SPF 4.

*With all sun screens, reapply every 2 hours.

MORE TIPS ON WRINKLE-FREE TANNING

- Everyone's skin is different and, therefore, may respond differently to the Tan Plan's guidelines . . . so it's important to *get to know when your tanning time is up*—that is, when your skin is just slightly pink, as if it were blushing.
- *Never go out in the sun with suntan oil or butter*—they provide no protection whatsoever.
- *If you're on the beach, move; don't just sit.* Your blood will circulate faster (thus better supplying your skin's cells with nutrients), and you'll receive less of a reflection from the sand.
- *Familiarize yourself with the sun's albedo*—the reflection of its rays off various surfaces. A good general way to gauge the sun's albedo is to keep in mind that black surfaces absorb the sun's rays while white, light surfaces reflect them. For example, powdery white beaches are extremely reflective, and even if you're under an umbrella you're still going to receive up to 50 percent of the sun's burning rays!

Surface	Sun's Albedo
snow	90%
water	50%
sand	40%
concrete	40%
grass	25%

- *Wear sunglasses*, preferably with brown or sage-green polarized lenses dark enough so that when you look in the mirror, you can not easily see your eyes through the lenses. (Skiers do best with amber lenses, which create a contrast to the snow.) Without sunglasses (or if yours aren't dark enough), you'll squint and end up with crow's-feet. Consider, too, photochromic lenses, which darken in bright light, and mirrored lenses, which reflect light away, keep you cool, too; both are good in glare conditions, such as sailing in summer, skiing in winter, but I don't recommend either as highly as the dark polarized lenses. And, always a good idea except for driving since they block peripheral vision: special eye guards (meant to block sun and wind) you can easily attach to your frames (they're part of Catherine's skiing ritual . . . plus she says she keeps her sunglasses on a string around her neck so they're always with her should the sun come out) or glasses that have special side pieces that are part of the lenses (below).

• *Use a bronzer to make a light tan darker—and safer.*

• *Exfoliate!* Dead skin cells can ruin a healthy glow, and prod you into getting darker than really necessary.

• *Beware of windburn.* On windy days, whether it's sunny or not, whether you burn easily or not, in both summer and winter, use a sun screen with SPF 15 or higher on exposed parts of your body. Wind not only intensifies sun's reaction, it can be extremely damaging as it breaks down the skin's oil barrier and whips away moisture, leaving skin dehydrated, flaky, itchy and rough. Be especially conscious of windburn in winter: Cold dry air blowing on the face causes skin to lose moisture at an accelerated rate.

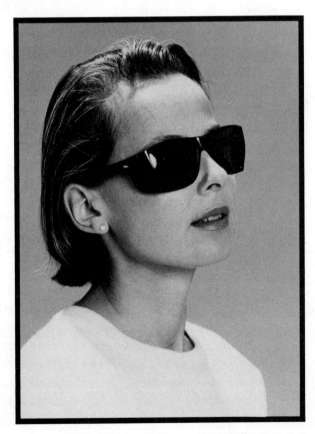

AND SHOULD YOU BURN . . .

No matter how diligent you are about following the Tan Plan, there may be times when you do burn, when, say, you miscalculate the sun's intensity or misread your tanning time—easy enough to do because sunburning may occur in as short a time as ten minutes, though its effects may not be visible for at least six hours.

What happens when you burn: The skin reddens, blood vessels swell, tissues break and, in serious cases, the damaged cells peel off, making way for newly produced cells, which upon immediate exposure are sensitive and extremely vulnerable. *When peeling occurs, do not go out into the sun for two days.* This will give skin the time it needs to regenerate, build up a new sun-resistant protective layer that is, in fact, harder and thicker (and, therefore, tougher-looking!) than the one that preceded it.

More Skin-Saving Remedies

Aspirin. Take two aspirins every four hours—they'll slow the workings of prostaglandin, a natural body chemical that helps produce sunburn, and they'll deaden the pain, too. Also, if you're sunburn prone, some experts believe taking two aspirins before sun exposure will not only deflect damage but may promote a better tan, too.

Cold compresses. To relieve pain and dissipate body heat, take a cool bath and apply cold milk compresses to burned areas—its lactic acid is healing. (Soak a washcloth in a bowl filled with ice cubes and equal parts of milk and water.)

Vitamin E. A lot of skin-care experts believe in the healing powers of vitamin E taken either orally or applied topically (just break open a capsule and apply).

Moisturizing. Invariably on a Monday morning early in July, I am faced with sunburned editors in desperate need of a moisturizer. What's happened is that in the time it's taken them to get to work, the moisturizer they applied before putting on makeup has been absorbed into the skin, leaving it feeling dry and parched again. The reason: Moisturizers don't last as long on sunburned skin as they do on normal skin, because sunburned skin is warmer and the warmth causes the rapid evaporation of not just the moisturizer itself but moisture in the skin, too. I usually give them a lightweight moisturizer so they can apply it throughout the day and not look (or feel) greasy.

Sunspot-fading products. Sometimes after overexposure to the sun, you may find dark spots on your skin. You can fade them with over-the-counter bleaching creams applied once or twice a day according to package instructions—and by minimizing sun exposure during treatment. If you don't see a lightening of the pigment within two months, see a dermatologist—the product isn't working for you. To prevent further "spotting," be sure your diet includes ample vitamin C and zinc.

HOW TO GET A SUNLESS SUNTAN

Here are a few great—and very natural-looking—ways to fake a tan. They're especially useful for sun-sensitive women . . . or during prolonged periods of poor weather.

- *With a moisturizer or foundation.* Now newly available: special sheer summer-weight moisturizers and foundations that are lightly tinted (some contain sun screens, too). Another option: a color wash in shades of bronze or rose.
- *With blush.* This is a tanning trick I concocted myself after watching makeup artist Pablo Manzoni at work. After putting on foundation, with a natural bristle brush (the fatter the better), apply powder blush where you naturally blush. Any doubt about where you blush? Next time you work out or you're out in the sun, look at your face and note where the color is—probably on your cheekbones, temples, under the arch on each brow, the tip of your nose and along the forehead (where you should be sure it blends and fades into the hairline—you don't want a band of color!). You could also use a cream blush: Use a damp sponge and apply to the same spots, pressing it into the skin; don't spread it or it'll blend right into the foundation. Or mix a little bronzing gel into your moisturizer.

  What color to use? What's most natural-looking, the color closest to the shade you naturally tan—probably brown-based colors like mauve, russet or burgundy; or, perhaps, a bronze with a hint of red. (Stay away from colors with too much orange in them; have you ever seen anyone tan a beautiful shade of apricot?)

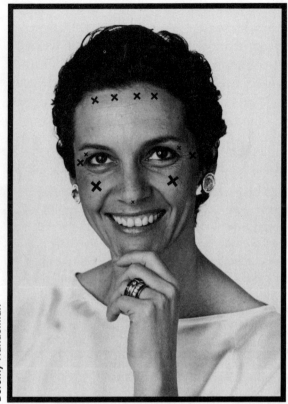

Dorothy Handelman

X marks the blush

With your "blush tan": Go for earth-tone eye shadows and a light lining of white on lower inside eye rim to make whites whiter; and, on lips, fruity colors (here's where you can use apricot or melon, a real red-orange coral).

> **For a great glow after dark: Brush a golden powder on cheeks, forehead, chin and earlobes.**

• *With self-tanning preparations.* Another way to fake a tan is with self-tanning lotions. They're especially good on pale, porcelainlike complexions for which makeup tans may look unnatural, or for seasonal firsts in a bathing suit.

Newly formulated in the last year or two, self-tanners no longer result in streaked yellow/orange colorings; now they're so natural-looking in color they can be mistaken for the real thing. Self-tanners react to certain amino acids in the upper layers of the skin. How dark your "tan" is depends on the amount of acids you have and on the number of applications, two or three usually providing a good rich color. Remember, your "tan" will last only as long as the skin's upper layers are intact; when they're shed, so your tan will be shed, and you'll need to reapply.

New now: the tanning pill, which also works as a sun screen on 50 percent of the people who take it. Currently available over the counter as Orobronze (Rorer) in Canada, France, Germany and Switzerland (but not yet in the U.S.), the tanning pill is made up of a food coloring that affects only the fatty part of the skin in the epidermis, turning it the same natural-looking golden-copper color you'd get after two or three days in the sun. Dosage is determined by weight (average 3–4 tablets a day)—too much turns the skin orange. It takes fifteen days for a tan to appear, and color lasts only as long as you continue taking the pill.

What about sun lamps? Tanning parlors? Stay away from them! When suntanning booths were first introduced in the seventies, they utilized UV-B, not UV-A, light and were criticized (and eventually became obsolete) because of the known risks of UV-B rays causing skin cancer, premature aging and eye damage. The new "safer" booths utilize UV-A, not UV-B rays. But, as I said earlier, though UV-A tans while UV-B burns, UV-A penetrates the dermis more deeply even than UV-B and thus causes severe damage and premature aging. In fact, UV-A exaggerates sunburning normally caused by UV-B light (thus the reason, if you stay under a sunlamp too long, you will burn!).

EIGHT

ANTIWRINKLE NEWS FROM THOSE IN THE KNOW

There are a number of professionals here and abroad whom I talk to regularly for the latest breakthroughs in skin care. They are the ones who always have the newest treatments and techniques, and the most useful and most effective tips for at-home care. For this book I asked each of them to select their newest de-aging salon/spa treatments and/or at-home tips. Coming right up, super antiwrinkle strategies from the best and the brightest in skin care ... some never before published! They're guaranteed to keep beautiful skin beautiful longer and to improve skin that's begun to show the signs of time. For addresses, phone numbers, see pages 219–26.

SKIN-ENHANCING STRATEGIES

Aromatherapeutic "Shock" Treatments: Diane Young Skin Care Center, New York City

Diane Young is among a handful of American believers in the European tradition of aromatherapy (that is, the use of essential oils and massage to treat the deep layers of the skin) to encourage new cell formation and to slow the aging process. One way to do this at home is to mix certain essential oils into a moisturizing facial mask to stimulate skin and shock it back into beautiful shape when it begins to show signs of aging. For broken capillaries and/or dry skin, she suggests chamomile, lavender or jasmine; for wrinkled, saggy skin, marigold, frankincense and orange blossom. You can find essential oils in health food stores. For more information, Diane recommends writing to Inner Traditions International, 377 Park Avenue South, New York, New York 10016.

Skin-Enhancing Treatment Baths: Canyon Ranch Spa, Tucson, Arizona

When we went to Canyon Ranch Spa, Catherine and I talked Deborah Morris, an herbalist, into giving us two of her favorite (and time-proven) antiwrinkle remedies to try at home.

The Vapor-Bath Facial (which many naturopaths believe is one of the best antiwrinkle remedies there is): In a large pot, boil about 6 quarts of water, and add 2 teaspoons fennel seeds per cup water. Let steep for 5 to 6 minutes. Cover your head with a big towel and steam your face for 20 minutes, maximum. When you're finished strain the fennel and mix a little of the liquid with honey or yogurt to form a paste. Apply to face. Leave on 20 minutes more and wash.

The Sweat Bath. Get your bathroom hot and steamy by running a hot shower for 5 to 10 minutes. Then fill the tub with hot-as-you-can-stand-it water. Soak for 20 minutes. Then—and this is important—when you get out of the tub, wrap yourself, head included, in towels and get into bed with three or four blankets (an electric blanket on top of that if you have one) for 20 minutes.

Though many people feel sweating is drying, according to Deborah, there's nothing like sweating for eliminating toxins from the skin, bringing up more natural oils to the surface. A word of caution: If you don't tolerate heat therapy well, if you feel faint in a whirlpool bath, sauna or steam room, this is not for you.

Antiaging Diet: Hippocrates Health Institute, Boston

One of the best-kept secrets among spa aficionados is the Hippocrates Health Institute in Boston, founded by Ann Wigmore, a Lithuanian who emigrated to the United States nearly sixty years ago when she was just sixteen. Though it's been around longer than many of the better-known spas, the twenty-year-old Hippocrates (as it's fondly referred to by its devotees) was new to both Catherine and me until quite recently.

After she arrived in the United States, Wigmore cured herself twice—once of gangrene, once of cancer—by eating garden grasses and weeds, which she calls youth food. Her spa plan is based on an antiaging diet. Her two main diet dos:

- Eat living foods that haven't been cooked, smoked, preserved or changed in any way from their natural state (Wigmore particularly advocates eating a lot of sprouts, since she believes they contain the most nutrients at germination time). Once they are tampered with (even cooked), foods lose not just their vitamins but their enzymes, which are necessary for assimilating vitamins in the body. "Dead" food, Wigmore holds, becomes sludge in the intestine, producing toxins as it decays and providing the perfect breeding ground for diseases to flourish.
- Every day drink at least one glass of chlorophyll-laden wheat grass juice to cleanse the blood and flood the body with vitamin E and precious enzymes. (To make: Soak wheat seeds in plain water for about 10 to 15 hours, draining and changing the water three times, until they sprout; then soak sprouts in filtered water (you need three times as much water as sprouted wheat) for 24 hours. Strain and drink. Note: You can store the sprouted wheat in the refrigerater and keep for another use.

Skin-tightening Paraffin Treatments: Christiana and Carmen Skin Care Salon, New York City

A mother-and-daughter team that cares for some of the most beautiful complexions in New York, Christiana and Carmen have found that their warm paraffin mask is one of the best "cures" for wrinkled skin.

The paraffin mask, which also includes super moisturizing ingredients such as azulene oil, is put on warm. The heat incites perspiration as it opens pores. But because the mask forms an occlusive seal on the surface of the skin, the fluids are reabsorbed by the skin, plumping wrinkles and smoothing the skin.

Lip-line Treatment: Georgette Klinger Skincare Salons; New York City, Beverly Hills, Dallas, Chicago, Bal Harbour, Palm Beach

Now, as part of a regular monthly facial she recommends for her clients, Miss Klinger includes a special lip treatment, which uses a concentrated gentle massage and a lubricating cream to soften existing lines, prevent them from deepening. Here's how to do the lip treatment at home in four easy steps (use your moisturizer and look into the mirror).

1. Purse lips. With your index fingers, massage upper lip area from the middle out, feeling your fingers moving your skin in the opposite direction of the "purse." Repeat 10 times.

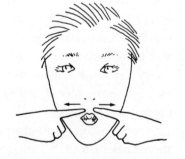

Margaret A. Hinders

2. Relax lips and press them together. With your index fingers, massage lower lip area from the middle out. Repeat 10 times.

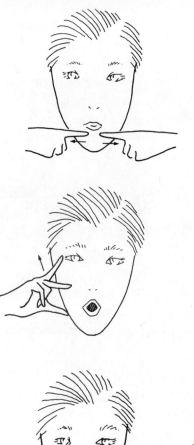

3. Make an O with lips. Take your right hand and place three fingers on the right side of your face: index finger at outer corner of right eye, middle finger on right cheekbone and thumb on chin under right cheek. Stroke with all three fingers up and out toward hairline. Repeat on left side.

4. Use forefingers to "iron" upper and lower lip areas. Do for 10 seconds on the upper lip, 10 seconds on the lower, too.

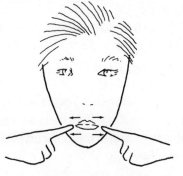

Margaret A. Hinders

The Bull Blood Wine Treatment and the Quail Egg Mask: Ilona of Hungary Institutes of Skin Care; New York City, Denver, Chicago, Houston

Named for the mineral-rich Hungarian wine that's one of its primary ingredients, the Bull Blood Wine Treatment utilizes an oxygenized cream formulated to oxygenate blood and thus stimulate cell regeneration as well as to encourage shedding of old cells and to rev up circulation.

Quail eggs, Ilona has discovered, are a super skin food, as they are readily absorbed and utilized to moisturize, nourish and condition. She simply whips together the yoke and the white, applies the "lotion" to a clean face and uses iontophoresis (indirect massage with a mild electric current) to induce deep penetration. To remove: She uses cotton saturated with herbal tea.

Wrinkle Ironing: Lia Schorr Skin Care, New York City

You iron wrinkles out of your clothes; well, Lia Schorr does the same on the face! After a light massage with a collagen cream, a tiny iron is warmed and gently smoothed across clients' lines. The warmth of the iron helps the cream penetrate the skin, softening and nourishing it, as it flattens the skin and forces the wrinkle into smoothness.

Scandinavian Brewer's Yeast Mask: Ole Henriksen of Denmark Skin Care Center, Los Angeles

Aware of brewer's yeast's antiaging benefits but also of its unpleasant taste, Ole Henriksen developed a special brewer's yeast mask he knows his clients will use to tone, tighten and de-age skin as well as to boost microcirculation to the face.

To make: Mix 2 tablespoons brewer's yeast powder, 1 egg white and 1 tablespoon apple juice (or mineral water, carbonated or not, it doesn't matter) until a thick paste forms. After a deep cleansing or after you've exfoliated, apply with upward and outward motions over entire face except for the eye area. (If you have normal/dry skin, apply over a moisturizer to prevent superficial dryness after the mask is removed; normal/oily skin types can apply the mask directly to their skin.) Lie down for 20 minutes; cover eyes with milk or tea compresses. Use three times a week. (See above.)

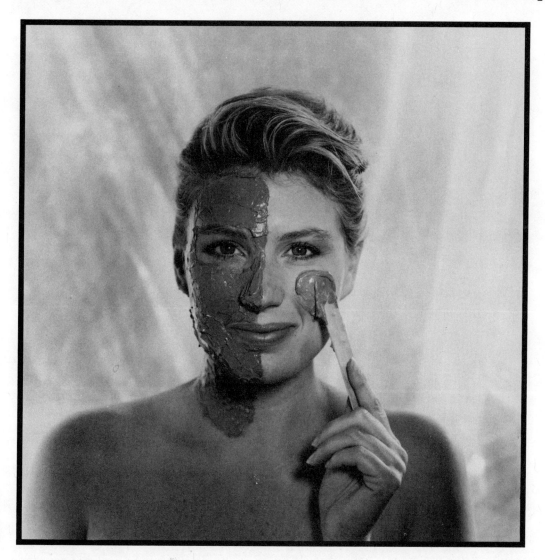

John Colao

Here, too, is Ole's special Eye Cream Formula: 1,200 IUs vitamin E (capsules); 50,000 IUs vitamin A (capsules); 2,500 IUs vitamin D (capsules); 2 teaspoons petroleum jelly, 1 teaspoon sesame or almond oil. Just squeeze contents from capsules and mix. Store in refrigerator and use morning and evening as needed.

Head-to-Toe Youthening: Panache Appearance Studios, Torrance, California

The philosophy here is that no single thing—not the best skin treatment or makeup job or hairstyle—will help you look well for your age. Good looks are a total package, and that's what owner Christine Kunzelman offers (complete transformation!) in her day-long "makeover." Included: a color analysis for clothes and makeup; a figure analysis for choosing proper clothing; a session in the art of accessorizing; skin-care–treatment analysis; a deep cleansing facial; hair-care recommendations including perming, coloring, cutting (whatever is necessary) and styling tips; a step-by-step makeup lesson, including eyebrow shaping.

Revitalizing Point System: Kerstin Skin Care, Laguna Beach, California

Swedish-born aesthetician Kerstin Florian has replaced the traditional facial massage with the beauty point system, which she recommends clients do at home at least two times a week, preferably daily. Based on the Chinese principle of acupuncture, the beauty point system applies gentle pressure at specific points of the face to relieve built-up tension. It takes about five minutes. Here's how she does it: First, she applies phytolene concentrate (a mixture of rosemary, lemon and organic silicone) to a clean face. (You can use your moisturizer.) Then, beginning at the forehead, moving down the nose to the chin, then up to cheeks, she presses gently but firmly with her middle finger in each of about fifteen spots for 5 seconds. The client inhales before pressure is applied, exhales while finger is on each beauty point.

One super skin rejuvenator from Kerstin: Combine 1 ounce wheat germ oil with 3 drops each of orange flower oil, sage oil, melissa oil, sweet marjoram oil and lavender oil (available at health food stores). Use 1 or 2 drops once or twice a week after a shower or bath when skin is warm (the warmth helps the cream penetrate).

Pincements Jacquet: Aida Thibiant Skin and Body Care Center, Beverly Hills, California

At night, after you apply your moisturizer, Aida Thibiant recommends pincements jacquet movements (a French term meaning the pinching of the skin between the thumbs and middle fingers) to boost blood circulation and help the cream penetrate the skin. Pinch your entire face and finish by tapping your chin and jaw with the back of your hand.

Bee Pollen and Shark-Liver Oil Treatments: Livia Sylva Bee Pollen Clinic de Beauté, New York City

The basis of Livia's antiwrinkle skin-rejuvenating plan is bee pollen gathered from flowers grown in a toxin-free, pollutant-free environment and imported from Romania. It comes in ampoule and tablet form.

Another of Livia's antiaging secrets: shark-liver oil, which she imports from France—it penetrates the skin and stimulates sluggish sebaceous glands to lubricate dry skin. Livia combines the oil with distilled water, propyglycol and iron powder to produce a thick cream, which she applies to the skin, lets dry, then removes with a special magnet.

Deep-pore Cleansing: Adriana's Skin Care, New York City

Romanian-born and -trained aesthetician Adriana Timus believes that nothing keeps skin younger- and healthier-looking than proper cleansing. Catherine has been going to Adriana for years and feels Adriana's deep-pore cleansing is largely responsible for keeping her skin young, smooth and firm. After one of Adriana's facials she says her pores look smaller, her complexion clearer, rosier. "No, you can't shrink pores, but it's logical that if your pores are clogged with dirt and grime they'll look larger, just like a soft suitcase bulges with an overload of clothes."

Adriana recommends a facial every four to six weeks for most of her clients and, in addition, four times a year, a special eye-hydrating mask: After a facial, when skin is receptive to the mask, Adriana smooths eye skin with a mask that moisturizes, makes tissues firmer and more supple.

Electric Wrinkle-removing "Facial": Christine Valmy's Skin Care Salons; New York City, Forest Hills, NY

A very fine needle through which galvanic currents travel is inserted at a 45-degree angle into the surface of the wrinkled skin. The current causes the skin's proteins to harden at the bottom of the line, lifting it and filling it out.

The treatment, which is usually done in four sessions (twice a week for two weeks) works beautifully on fine lines around the eyes and lips and on the forehead. Treatments have to be repeated at regular six- to eight-week intervals (because the hardened skin protein is eventually pushed away by the skin's natural renewal process). It is totally painless.

Oxygenation Facial and Skin-tightening Peel: Aida Grey Institut de Beauté, Beverly Hills

To regenerate surface skin cells, Aida Grey treats clients to her Progressive Moisturized Oxygenation Facial, which utilizes oxygenated steam and a moisturizing serum extracted from vegetables. For best results she recommends the regenerating facial after a special chemical peeling treatment: The chemical, left on the skin for 1½ hours, is removed with carefully prepped cotton pads; the actual peeling takes place over the next seven days. Benefits (better texture and tone) last up to two years.

At-home Yogurt Mask: Klisar Skin Care Center, New York City

Super hydrating and revitalizing for older skin: the yogurt mask. Mix 4 ounces plain yogurt with 1 tablespoon calcium carbonate (available in health food stores) and 2 tablespoons calimium powder until you get a smooth consistency. Apply to entire face except eye and throat areas (use a cream on both these areas). Lie down for ten to fifteen minutes with two pieces of cucumber on eyes, legs elevated on a pillow. Rinse with tepid water; moisturize.

Skin Pickups: T. J. D'Ifray Institut de Beauté, Beverly Hills

Judith D'Ifray sent me information on her Volcanic Ash Mask, which, she said, mixed with herbs, milk and honey, reduces the appearance of wrinkles dramatically. We started talking, and I felt she had a wealth of unique ideas about skin care. Here, a sampling:

- Use your pinkies (because they exert so little pressure) to apply treatment products to eye and mouth areas; middle and index fingers on the rest of the face; the palm of hand on neck.
- Wipe away moisturizer residue after 20 minutes—by then it's done what it's going to do.
- Exfoliate the skin with gentle gelatin peeler: Add about 3 teaspoons water to a packet of gelatin, apply paste to skin, let dry and remove immediately. Rinse with warm water; apply moisturizer.
- Soothe puffy eyes with chamomile tea bags you've moistened with boiling water, then stored in the freezer so they're ready to use when you need them.

Cell Revitalization Therapy: Peter Stephan's Center, London

A disciple once removed of La Prairie's Paul Niehans (his late father worked with Niehans—see p. 184), Peter Stephan has refined and perfected the science of cellular regeneration (that is, giving aging bodies live cells from newly slaughtered unborn lambs). Stephan uses injections or suppositories of organ-specific RNA—say, liver RNA to strengthen a damaged liver.

Though the injections or suppositories aren't specifically for aging skin, they do rejuvenate skin, Stephan says, because skin is a mirror of what goes on inside your body . . . and healthy internal organs mean healthy, young skin, too.

Bonus! Soon available in the United States: Stephan's newly developed treatment cream formulated from skin serum (connective tissue, blood vessels and muscle) that restores, softens and plumps the upper layer of the skin, prevents the formation of lines.

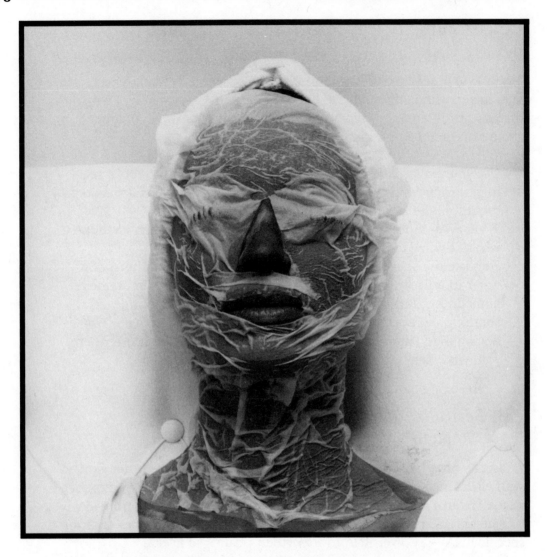

Caviar! Beauty Food: Ingrid Millet Institut de Beauté; Paris, New York City

In Paris and New York, at Ingrid Millet's Institut de Beauté, caviar isn't just for eating. It's for nourishing the skin, too. The reason: While human skin has a positive charge, live-cell marine products—caviar among them (Millet also uses sea mud masks)—have negative charges. So, when the caviar treatment is applied to the skin (above), its nourishing elements (potassium, magnesium and niacin) are drawn by osmosis into the skin and, as they penetrate to the live cells beneath the epidermis, they plump the skin cells, smooth away lines, produce an unmistakable beauty blush.

Foot Reflexology: Laura Norman and Associates, New York City

I couldn't have been more skeptical when I first heard about it: Foot reflexology, the application of pressure to certain points on your feet that correspond to different organs, glands and muscles in your body, is supposed to induce relaxation, eliminate tension and tension-produced wrinkles and increase circulation. I was skeptical about the whole science until Laura Norman, M.S., a certified reflexologist and licensed massage therapist, came to my office to give me a minitreatment (a 15-minute version of the full 50-minute one she usually gives patients).

I was absolutely amazed: After a few minutes of Laura's pressing, kneading and rubbing, I began to feel my body warm and relax. I felt my shoulders drop, my facial muscles untense. I began to doze. I was sold. Of course I didn't look years younger afterward, but I certainly looked more relaxed, and I can see how a series of treatments could benefit my skin (and my psyche!).

Here's why: The deep relaxation releases the stress that causes some wrinkles and eases the tightness in the neck and shoulders that cuts off blood flow to the face. In addition, it cleans up dark undereye circles and it improves proper elimination of wastes (the kidney and eye zones are the same point in the foot).

Why is a foot massage better than a facial or a neck massage? Laura says direct massage can enhance tension (some people tense up when someone works close to their face; the feet represent a "safe" distance, she says). Also, because of the pull of gravity, working the feet, unlike working the face and neck, gets the blood flow going back up to the face.

Tip: Drink a large glass of water after each treatment to further flush away toxins.

Like any massage, the benefits of foot reflexology are best felt when it's done by a pro. However, here are Laura's step-by-step instructions for giving yourself a 10-minute treatment.

- Sit in a comfortable position in a quiet room.
- Place the thumb of one hand on the heel of the opposite foot and, using a light, absorbent, greaseless lotion, use steady, even pressure to press point by point up to the base of toes. (This is called thumb walking.)
- Then do the top of your feet, using your fingers. (This is called finger walking.)
- Last, concentrate on the big toe, which corresponds to the head and face.

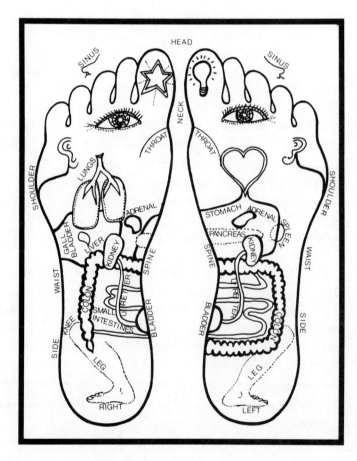

NEWS! THE NATURAL APPROACH TO DE-AGING

Phytochemistry (plant cosmetology) has grown in the last decade from kitchen remedies to a practical, respectable science. Plants have a natural chemical affinity to skin and they're being recommended by many experts (as you now know) for use on their own, too. Following, some of the most popular . . . and why they're making big beauty news.

Sea Food for Older Skin

Seawater and seaweed (or sea algae) are chock full of rejuvenating nutrients that moisturize older skin, make it more elastic, stronger, younger-looking. Seawater, whose composition is almost identical to blood plasma, is composed of about 35 percent minerals and salts (regular water, only 7 percent); and seaweed is really just superconcentrated seawater (about ten times richer).

Look for moisturizers, body lotions, masks and shampoos containing seawater and algae. Or: (1) Chop some seaweed and simply position it on your face while you lie down for 20 minutes; and (2) sun-dry seaweed and store in a plastic bag; for a deep-pore cleansing, mix it with a cream cleanser and massage into face; rinse well.

Note: Mineral-rich sea mud is therapeutic and is used in many spas: There are mud baths, head-to-toe mud masks and facial masks.

Clay

Rich in natural minerals that draw impurities from the skin, clay is particularly good for older skin because as it absorbs cellular debris, it tightens pores and stimulates circulation in the uppermost layers of the skin, leaving you with a healthy, rosy glow.

Clay is commonly used as a cleansing mask, and because it works so efficiently, often drying the skin, take special care to choose the kind of clay that's best for your skin type: If you have oily skin, go for dark brown, mudlike clays or green clay (which can also be used for combination skin); if you have sensitive or dry skin, go for white clay, which is extremely gentle; rose clay is good for all types of skin, even sensitive.

> Tip for home treatments: When you use natural ingredients (milk, yogurt, etc.), only use freshly made preparations, never leftovers—you'll only reap benefits if the living substances have not oxidized due to exposure to air.

Bee Pollen

Some say it's the fountain of youth: Bee pollen is said to prevent premature aging of skin cells, stimulate growth of new cells, protect against dehydration . . . and smooth away wrinkles!

In a study conducted by a Swedish dermatologist, Lars-Erik Essen, M.D., patients who used pollen cream showed smoother, healthier, rosier skin: Forehead wrinkles decreased in depth—they didn't totally disappear—as did lines around the eyes (though they took longer than forehead furrows).

Aloe Vera

A great natural ingredient known for its face-saving properties is aloe vera. It moisturizes beautifully (aloe gel itself is 97 percent water) and helps skin fight bacteria.

Many products contain aloe vera, or you can easily grow your own. Make sure that what you have is an aloe vera plant; there are about 200 species. When you want to use it simply break off a leaf (the plant will reseal itself) and squeeze to extract the gel—a few drops on the face will keep it well moisturized.

THE ANTIAGING SUPER SPAS

Spas have been popular in Europe for years, and only in the last decade or so have they begun popping up in the United States—and they're catching on fast, especially now that women are working (spas are the perfect hassle-free getaway for women on their own). A week at a spa can do wonders for relieving stress, providing a good (and beautifying) rest.

Among all the spas around the world, there are a handful that I feel can take years off your looks (in addition to everything else they do). Here they are . . . and what they offer that's de-aging.

Here in the United States and Mexico . . .

• At *The Ashram Health Resort* in Calabasas, California, the emphasis is on de-aging attitudes about chronological age, "refocusing on biological age." How it's done: a rigorous exercise schedule and a vegetarian diet limited to just 600 calories a day stretch guests to their physical limits and so effect a change in attitude about oneself and life in general.

• *Canyon Ranch Spa*, Tucson, Arizona, bases its program on the theory of "wellness"—that is, taking responsibility for your own health and good looks. At the ranch there's every opportunity to do so: Available right there are nutritionists; biofeedback therapists; skin-care, makeup, hair-care and fitness experts. Plus, for those guests who are considering plastic or reconstructive surgery, the ranch is affiliated with a board-certified plastic surgeon who's available for chemical peels as well as more major surgery.

• At *The Golden Door* in Escondido, California, you'll be pampered like never before. This is the ultimate spa, the spa of spas, for head-to-toe de-aging. The emphasis is on natural skin-saving foods, deliciously prepared and served in quantities ranging from 700 to 2000 calories a day; fitness combined with relaxing herbal wraps, saunas, massages and wrinkle-removing facials; complete privacy and peace; and developing a whole new way of caring for yourself. And all this in beautifully designed Japanese-inspired facilities with an employee-guest ratio of three to one! The Golden Door just can't be beat.

• *Rancho La Puerta*, Tecate, Baja California, Mexico, the precursor of The Golden Door (both are owned and run by Deborah Szekely), is the biggest health resort in North America—and probably the best place for relaxing and rejuvenating with the whole family. The ranch program centers on a vegetarian diet (800 to 850 low-sodium, low-cholesterol calories a day)—and from Chapter 6 you know how good that can be for your skin. The food served is simple and fresh—so fresh, in fact, that many of the organic foods in the diet are raised right on the ranch, while many of the herbs used as seasonings are picked on surrounding hillsides. There's also an emphasis on rigorous exercise—everything from aerobic exercise classes to tennis, swimming and yoga.

• If you're looking for a spa where an all-day vigorous workout is not de rigueur, *Maine Chance*, Phoenix, Arizona, may be just the place for you—here you are de-aged in extravagant (and relaxing) luxury. However, should the spirit move you, there is a 90-minute daily exercise regimen that, combined with the 900-calorie-a-day diet, is guaranteed to help you lose weight.

. . . And Abroad

• European aging cures have been a step (or more) ahead of ours for years, and when I was at *Clinic La Prairie*, Montreux, Switzerland, in 1980, it was almost the first I'd heard of cellular renewal in anything but the most abstract terms. And today La Prairie's therapy is extremely advanced.

The clinic's founder, the late Dr. Paul Niehans, used injections of young healthy cells taken from fetal lambs to stimulate cell growth in the human body. The same treatment is being used today (very successfully!)—and what this means for the patient is better circulation, improved skin elasticity, even all-around increased energy. La Prairie recommends thirty-five to forty-five as the optimum age to start treatment (this involves a one-week stay). Doing so then will retard the aging process and, in fact, may even avert the need for a face-lift altogether. *Note:* This is not a "fancy" spa. It is, as its name implies, a clinic, which can accommodate twenty-four patients a week.

• The draw at *Terme di Montecatini* in the hills of Tuscany is water—thermal water, that is. You can take the hydroponic therapy (drinking the waters—there are five and each one treats a different bodily function); balneotherapy (thermal baths); hydrotherapy (showers); and fangotherapy (mud baths and compresses). The spring water is alkaline, predominantly sodium-chloride-sulfate, and, according to the rich and famous who come here from all over the world for fifteen to twenty days of treatments, is said to be extremely effective in rejuvenating, inside and out.

• *Quiberon Institute*, Brittany, France, is the leader in thalassotherapy (sea therapy) in France. Two 10-day cures a year—they include saltwater and/or seaweed baths, seawater whirlpool baths, sea mud body and face masks, exercise classes, swimming in the Olympic-size saltwater pool—can take ten years off your looks.

• On *The Gerovital Treatment Tours* in Romania, professor Ana Aslan uses procaine-based Gerovital H3 (injections and pills) to counteract the effects of aging, improve bodily functions as well as arthritis, neuritis and asthma. Treatment takes fourteen days, but after you receive your prescription in Bucharest, you can travel to doctor-staffed clinics around Romania to continue treatment.

• More Gerovital H3 treatments at the *Spa at the Hotel Plantation de Leyritz* on Martinique in the French West Indies: It's the same Romanian rejuvenator in another locale, perhaps not so far from home.

• Aesthetician Madame Alma Filion believes that wrinkles are caused by the skin's inability to slough off dry and/or dead cells, and, at *The Filion Spa* in Toronto, Ontario, she's come up with an exfoliator that not only does this but rejuvenates new cells in the process.

Humanly compatible enzymes taken from the stomachs of pigs (because their enzymes are strong) and lambs (because their enzymes rarely cause allergic reactions) are processed into dehydrated powder form; then they're mixed with oatmeal and hot water (which reactivates them) and are applied to the skin. Afterward, a skin soother that stops the action of the enzymes is put on the face, followed by a neutralizing cream that's used for two days to doubly ensure that enzyme action has stopped.

NINE

NONSURGICAL

FACE-LIFTS

I am not opposed to plastic surgery, but I do feel that in the past few years nonsurgical face-saving treatments have been developed and perfected to such an extent that you can delay surgery for ten or more years—and, in some cases, avoid it altogether. Coming up: your best options. Some have never been published before!

CHOOSING A GOOD SKIN DOCTOR

Finding an experienced and qualified doctor is often a lot easier said than done—and, in fact, one of the most common requests I get is to help friends and/or readers find a really good doctor. So I asked Barry Weintraub, M.D., a Beverly Hills plastic surgeon, for a step-by-step approach to the task. Here's what he told me.

Begin at the Beginning

There are three primary sources that'll provide you with names: (1) a local medical doctor—your family physician or your internist or gynecologist; (2) the American Society of Plastic and Reconstructive Surgeons Referral Service, 233 North Michigan Avenue, Suite 1900, Chicago, Illinois 60601, (312) 856-1834; or the American Academy of Dermatology, P. O. Box 3116, Evanston, Illinois 60204, (312) 869-3954; and (3) former patients.

Checking Credentials

Once you gather a few names, check to find out if the doctor has completed a bona fide educational residency in plastic surgery or dermatology, and if he or she is board certified, which means passing a series of exams representing the highest level of scrutiny by peers. To do: See if the doctor has the requisite diplomas on the wall and/or call the appropriate society/academy (listed earlier).

Have a Consultation

Everything check out? Go for a consultation. Are you comfortable talking with the doctor? Is he or she listening? Does he or she seem to be interested and concerned? Or abrupt and in a hurry? Is he or she willing to explain your options and discuss the details of each procedure, review its risks and possible complications as well as the recuperation period so you'll know how much time you might be out of work and how you'll look immediately afterward? If so, does the doctor seem knowledgeable and experienced? Does he or she make any recommendations, ask for (or show you) photos to determine what seems aesthetically pleasing to you? With answers to all of these questions, you should be ready—and able—to make an educated, intelligent decision.

THE SILICONE VS. COLLAGEN CONTROVERSY

Ever since its approval by the FDA in 1981, injectable collagen has been getting a great deal of press—but still, I find there's a lot of confusion about it (what it does, how it works, how it differs from silicone, its pros, its cons . . . and more). It is, I'd say, the subject of more than half the questions I receive from readers, friends and friends of friends, many of whom still don't realize that *collagen doesn't require surgery—it's an injection!—and it doesn't require any recuperation time* or time off from work. In fact, you can have it done on a lunch hour!

Here's my position on injectable collagen: After an endless number of interviews with doctors on both the research and clinical sides of collagen applications, I'd say that with very few exceptions collagen injections are the safest, quickest, easiest and most painless and most foolproof and dramatic way of getting rid of wrinkles (actually, what it does is fill in wrinkles, not eliminate them—but it looks like they're gone and that's what counts!).

And its technology, which in just a few short years has already undergone advances, is always improving. The new Zyderm II collagen is substantially more efficient in certain areas (deeper folds, frown lines) than Zyderm I (most efficient around the eyes), since it has 65 percent collagen as compared to I's 35 percent. What this means is that the two Zyderms can be used to complement one another for maximum effectiveness.

Many doctors recommend collagen over silicone: The American Society of Plastic and Reconstructive Surgeons, Inc., recommends that silicone, because of the number of complications it seems to incur, should not be used except for severe congenital deformities that can't be helped in any other way. And, in fact, the Food and Drug Administration has never approved the use of silicone except in the hands of a few select doctors who have had years of experience with it. (If you do decide to use it, be absolutely sure that the doctor injecting it is one of the few sanctioned by the FDA.)

I contacted the American Society of Plastic and Reconstructive Surgeons, Inc., to get their most up-to-date stance on silicone. This is what they told me:

> The American Society of Plastic and Reconstructive Surgeons, in cooperation with Dow Corning Corporation, who manufactures liquid silicone, has established strict guidelines under the auspices of the federal Food and Drug Administration for the judicious use of this agent in clinical trials. As you may be aware, there have been reports of complications from the alleged injection of "liquid silicone" of unknown manufacturing sources. The use of this fluid in the breast is absolutely contraindicated and is discouraged for wrinkles at present. However, for specifically severe deformities of the facial area, liquid silicone may be acceptable treatment.
>
> Therefore, the Dow Corning Corporation, in cooperation with the federal Food and Drug Administration and the American Society of Plastic and Reconstructive Surgeons, has designated certain clinical in-

vestigators to use this drug with patients in specific categories. All data collected from the investigation was compiled in the latter part of 1981 and submitted to the federal Food and Drug Administration for study. [So you can see, the verdict on silicone is still not in.]

For your own safety, we wish to warn you that many of the problems that are alleged to be treated easily with liquid silicone can be treated by other means, which have passed the test of time as safe and effective. There is no officially recognized source of medical grade liquid silicone, except that available to the investigators through the Dow Corning Corporation. Therefore, you should be warned not to seek liquid silicone from physicians other than the investigators.

Here's why, very simply, collagen is better than silicone, according to Craig Foster, M.D., a New York City plastic surgeon.

- Collagen is a natural protein, purified and sterilized, made from calf hide and so similar to human collagen it's easily integrated into the dermis of the skin and actually becomes a lifelike fabric of your skin. Silicone, on the other hand, is a foreign body; it is a synthetic substance that is never really accepted by the body. In actuality, a tissue reaction forms around the implant, "walling" it off from the rest of the body.
- Collagen wears away (as does your natural collagen). Though this could be viewed as a negative (many women want one shot that'll last a lifetime), it is, in fact, a real plus: Should there be any negative reactions to collagen, they go away within three to five days, and any that linger longer, within the next couple of weeks. Silicone, on the other hand, is for forever—and so, too, are some of its possible complications (including inflammatory responses and, after a number of years, glossy skin and a diminishing of surface contours).
- Collagen requires a board-certified plastic surgeon or dermatologist, to be sure, but silicone even more so, because the wrong doctor with wrong technique will cause permanent damage. And no matter how good a doctor is, he's only human—and fallible. The bottom line: Collagen allows for a greater margin of error than silicone.
- Collagen is injected superficially—and painlessly—right under the surface of the skin. Silicone is a subcutaneous filling that must be injected deep in the dermis.

· Collagen stays put. Silicone has been known to move from the injection site. (In addition, what may happen is that as you age and your skin thins, the correction that was perfect when you were 35 is an over-correction at 50. And you can see the ridge of silicone!)
· With collagen, especially the new highly concentrated Zyderm II, you'll see results after one to two treatments. With silicone, it takes six office visits to see results, because the substance must be injected in microdroplets.

News! A brand-new (improved!) injectable collagen has been introduced by the Collagen Corporation, makers of Zyderm I and II. The Zyplast Implant provides extra stability, expanding the uses of injectable collagen to include deeper lines; firmer, thicker scars; and even contour deformities.

COLLAGEN

How It Works

First, the skin test. To determine possible allergic reactions to collagen, a test dose is injected into the forearm about a month before treatment. Less than 3 percent of all patients show any sensitivity to the material (an allergic reaction will show reddening and swelling at the site), and they are not candidates for the treatment. (Another 1 percent become positive after the second test injection, which I would recommend even though a lot of doctors require only one test.) People with personal histories of autoimmune diseases, and anaphylactoid reactions (i.e., those with shortness of breath) and hypersensitivity to lidocaine (the local anesthetic in the collagen mixture) are also not collagen candidates.

Extra caution is taken with people who have histories of atopic or allergic reactions to other substances, who are getting immunosuppressive therapy, who have active inflammatory skin conditions such as cysts, pimples, rashes and hives, and with infections not under control. To date, the safety of the product with regard to pregnant women, infants and children has not been established.

Second, injecting the face-lift. Injectable collagen, suspended in a saline solution, is an odorless, whitish substance with the consistency of a soft gel that is injected with a fine-gauge needle into the wrinkle, filling it as it replaces the collagen lost due to your own tissue breakdown. The result: The depression is elevated to the same level as that of the surrounding skin, diminishing the wrinkle. Usually two to four injections are needed (spaced at least two weeks apart) to achieve maximum correction, but this varies with each patient.

"You can never predict with 100 percent certainty just how each patient will metabolize collagen and how it's going to wear," Dr. Foster told me. One thing is for certain, though: The thicker the skin, the less effective the results, because it's harder to flatten the wrinkle. Thus (and this is very general, since you can't assume thick skin is endemic to all peoples of certain races), Mediterraneans, blacks and hispanics are less likely to benefit from collagen injections than fair, thin-skinned Nordic types. People with sun-damaged skin, according to Dr. Foster, are good candidates.

After the injection, a slight (but not the least bit unsightly) swelling occurs; most of this subsides within twenty-four hours as the saline solution is absorbed by the body. Because the collagen is injected right under the surface of the skin, it can cause some lumping and ridging, sometimes whiteness and usually some soreness at the injection site. Whatever residual effects of the injections persist after the three- to five-day period will disappear completely in about four weeks (the longest in Dr. Foster's experience being seven to eight weeks).

You shouldn't go out in the sun for one month after treatments because sun breaks down injectable collagen (and the results will be diminished) just as it breaks down your own.

A small number of people (about 1 in 100) do experience more serious redness, swelling, firmness and itching at the injection site. Most of these reactions (half occur when reactions to the skin test are not noticed or reported and half occur if collagen was administered in spite of negative reactions to the skin test) last for between two weeks and four months, though some have lasted longer. In addition, about 1 in 1,000 patients develop an infection or a recurrence of herpes simplex. Some patients (fewer than 3 in 1,000) report nausea, achiness, headaches, dizziness and breathing difficulties; and some (fewer than 1 in 10,000) get a scab at the injection site (as a result of vessel laceration) that can result in scarring.

Third, the touch-up injections. Because collagen correction is not permanent (to reiterate, the injected collagen is so similar to your own that it, too, wears away in time), touch-ups are usually necessary twenty-four months after the original treatment (and every twenty-four months thereafter).

Recuperation Time

None.

Results

Here's what collagen can fix, what it can't.

COLLAGEN CAN FIX

- forehead furrows (if you use your forehead constantly, collagen will wear quickly)
- vertical wrinkles between brows
- fine creases at corners of eyes
- fine creases under eyes
- smile lines
- vertical wrinkles above and below lips
- droopy mouth (downward wrinkles at the corners of mouth)
- thinning lips
- lateral lines on chin
- harsh contours and depressions

COLLAGEN CAN'T FIX

- horizontal wrinkles above lips
- crosshatched skin
- double chin
- deep ice-pick acne scars

Recommendations/Risks

Another of collagen's plusses is that it is for everyone—for the thirty-year-old who doesn't really need a face-lift but who has lines she doesn't want to live with until she's old enough for plastic surgery; for anyone forty or over who wants to get rid of lines but who has an aversion to plastic surgery; and for those who've had surgery but still have lines they want touched up.

Disappearing Lines: The Collagen Correction

Suzanne Callaway (below) is a great example of how well collagen works for women in their late thirties (she's thirty-seven): Too young for plastic surgery, she felt she looked older than her years . . . and she was unhappy about it. We suggested collagen—and you can see how well it worked.

We sent her to Dr. Allyn Landau, who uses collagen not just to fill in lines but as a kind of soft contouring for skin that's beginning to sag (due to loss of subcutaneous fat) . . . and even where it isn't (just as a cosmetic boost). Here's what she did for Suzanne:

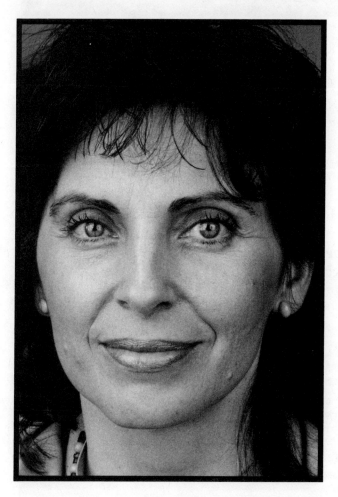

Before collagen injections

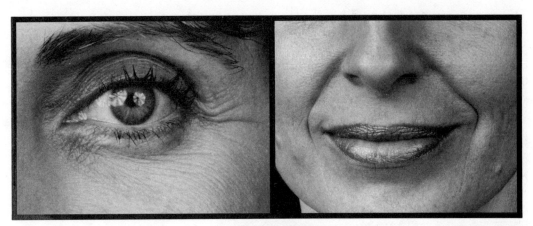

Key problem areas

- She filled in Suzanne's forehead furrows as well as her crow's-feet, fine lines between the brow and those under her eyes, which, she felt, when eliminated, would create a happier (younger-looking) face.
- Where Suzanne was starting to show some hollowness low in her cheeks (due to loss of estrogen), Dr. Landau used a few drops of collagen to fill in.
- Suzanne's lips were beginning to lose some of their definition and, even though it wasn't a major problem, Dr. Landau used a bit of collagen to make them slightly fuller, sexier.
- As for Suzanne's laugh lines: Though they were aging, as you can see in the before photo, those lines gave her a very interesting, chiseled look. So Dr. Landau used collagen to actually build up the lines at an angle (rather than fill them in completely) in order not to completely eliminate that unique feature.

The final touches: We wanted to show Suzanne how to make the most of her new younger look, so we asked Craig Gadson to help her with her makeup (you can see that he used a very light natural makeup, since she has fewer lines and needs less of a camouflage job) and to Gad Cohen to show her how to style her hair. He, too, went for a youthful natural look, held now off the face by mousse and spray.

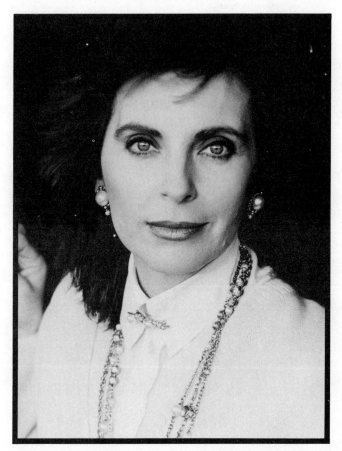

Suzanne's new "lift"

THE NEW WRINKLE FIBER—FIBREL

In the instance that collagen doesn't work, you have another equally good option: fibrel injections. Fibrel, a substance that stimulates the body's own collagen production, has been used successfully for several years to elevate depressed scars and is now being tested for filling in wrinkles also. It's a good alternative for those who are allergic to collagen (and it may be longer-wearing, too), because you are injecting the wrinkles with your own blood. The only reason I call it an alternative—and recommend collagen first—is that it is still being tested as a wrinkle filler . . . but, so far, Gary Monheit, M.D., a Birmingham, Alabama, dermatologist tells me, findings are very encouraging.

How It Works

The same amount of blood that's drawn for a blood test is taken from the patient and is "spun" down until just the serum remains. The serum is then mixed with an absorbable "filling" gelatin and the enzyme aminocaproic acid, which stimulates collagen production, making more than is normally needed. This three-part substance is injectable fibrel.

Recuperation Time

None. There's no risk of swelling or infection.

Results

Same as collagen, with one exception: Unlike collagen, fibrel can fill in deep ice-pick scars. Also—and this is very important—because fibrel is thicker than collagen, it may last longer. That means fewer initial injections and fewer touch-ups later.

Recommendations/Risks

Because fibrel is thicker than collagen, it requires a larger needle and, therefore, a local anesthetic. As with collagen, a patch test is done, but because your own blood is used, there is less chance of an allergic reaction.

THE MUSCLE-RELAXING INJECTABLE FOREHEAD LIFT

This is another injectable lift . . . but this one is so new only its "inventor," Stephen Genender, M.D., a Los Angeles plastic surgeon, and his associates, are doing it. "I haven't even discussed it with other plastic surgeons," Dr. Genender told me. But after six months of doing the procedure, he says the results are startling. The potential—both in terms of cosmetic and preventive applications—is phenomenal.

How It Works

Dr. Genender injects a toxin into wrinkle-forming muscles (usually on the forehead) to weaken them and so eliminate the wrinkle. (It's the same toxin ophthalmologists use to weaken the strong eye muscle that causes a child's eye to wander. Dr. Genender thought of using the toxin for wrinkles after reading about it in an ophthalmic journal.) The toxin doesn't destroy the muscle; it simply interferes to keep it from contracting—perfect, according to Dr. Genender, who had been looking for an alternative solution to cutting muscles (common in plastic surgery), because cut muscles reattach, and eventually frown lines come back.

Injections take a matter of seconds. Some areas require more than one—like the forehead (it takes about four)—but all are done at the same time, not in a series. There's very slight discomfort—an instantaneous burning, as if a local anesthetic were being injected, then nothing—that comes from the toxin itself, not the needle.

Recuperation Time

None. There's no risk of swelling or infection. To date, there have been no side effects whatsoever.

Results

These injections are extremely effective in smoothing deep forehead furrows and wrinkles between brows as well as crow's-feet. The muscle usually starts to weaken within forty-eight hours and is completely weakened in a week to ten days. Very deep established lines don't go away completely—immediately; but they are markedly diminished right away and, over a period of about a month, they do gradually disappear. As of now, Dr. Genender is using just enough toxin to last six months. It could be done to last one year.

In addition to smoothing existing lines, these injections can be used preventively wherever expression lines may form, Dr. Genender says.

Recommendations/Risks

Whether you consider this lift for cosmetic or preventive purposes, understand it's not a lift for loose, saggy skin—only for wrinkles.

The only negative result Dr. Genender has seen is that in a small percentage of patients, the toxin doesn't work and a second treatment is required. "If someone doesn't see complete results in two weeks, I just reinject them," he says. Any problem of having too much toxin? "Absolutely not. It's rapidly absorbed into the body."

DERMABRASION

An extreme form of exfoliation, dermabrasion actually removes the entire epidermis and upper portion of the dermis (about a third of your skin). Done by an experienced plastic surgeon or dermatologist—the art (and visual success of the procedure) lies in determining exactly the right depth of skin to remove for the particular skin type—dermabrasion is a safe, controllable, mechanical process that can be extremely effective, especially on faces that need resurfacing.

How It Works

For a full-face dermabrasion, general anesthesia may be administered. For a partial-face dermabrasion (say, on the mouth area), the skin is temporarily numbed with either a topical or a local anesthetic. But regardless of the type of anesthesia, the treatment is painless. A high-speed electrical device called a dermabrader is used to remove the upper layers of damaged skin, smooth wrinkles (especially weather lines, vertical lip lines and forehead lines), pockmarks, old scars, rough spots and brown spots. The whole procedure, which can be done in a doctor's office, takes one to one and a half hours.

Recuperation Time

There's a seven- to ten-day recuperation period. Plasma can ooze for a couple of days. Dr. Weintraub advises lukewarm showering on the second post-treatment day and each morning thereafter. Antibacterial ointment should be applied after each washing and, on about the seventh day, fresh, pink skin will appear. Hypoallergenic makeup and skin-care products designed especially for sensitive skin can be used on about the tenth posttreatment day. And don't go in the sun for two to four months after the treatment, because the new skin is highly susceptible to burning and pigmentary changes.

Results

The natural noticeable effects of dermabrasion—dramatically smoother, younger-looking skin!—can last for up to ten years!

Recommendations/Risks

Dermabrasion is best done on the whole face. If only a portion is done, it can make other wrinkled areas look worse. The procedure is particularly effective on uneven skin tones and/or on skin that has a leathery texture, crosshatching and sun damage. There is a risk of blotchy pigmentary changes, especially in dark- or olive-complected people. (In fact, it's not advisable for Orientals or blacks, because their pigment is so volatile.)

CHEMICAL PEELING

The procedure involves the use of a chemical solution that actually burns off the upper layer of skin. As with any burning process, it can be difficult to control. Therefore, proper application is critical and should be done by an experienced plastic surgeon or dermatologist.

How It Works

First, the skin is cleansed with acetone to remove extraneous debris and residual skin oils. After the induction of either local or general anesthesia, the solution is neatly applied to the skin using a cotton-tip applicator. This is done slowly, taking great care to monitor the patient's heart rhythm, because the chemical enters the bloodstream and tissues. Shortly after the solution is applied, the skin will take on a whitish, powdery appearance. In areas where there are particularly deep wrinkles, surgical tape can be applied to effect an even deeper peel. Chemical peeling works best on fine wrinkles, especially around the mouth, cheeks and forehead. According to Dr. Weintraub, chemical peeling is a "godsend," especially for women with vertical wrinkles on the upper and/or lower lip. This procedure, which is painless, takes up to one hour, depending on the extent of surface area to be peeled.

Recuperation Time

There is a seven- to ten-day recuperation period. As with dermabrasion, Dr. Weintraub recommends lukewarm showering on the second posttreatment day and each morning thereafter, and antibacterial ointment applications after each washing; makeup can be applied by the tenth postoperative day. There should be no direct prolonged sun exposure for two to four months after treatment. Later, during extended exposure to ultraviolet light, a sun screen should always be applied.

Results

The results in well-chosen patients can be nothing less than spectacular. They last for at least ten years.

Recommendations/Risks

Though chemical peeling can be effective on fine lines and wrinkles and on uneven skin tones, it is not a solution for deep expression lines or acne scars—it treats low and high skin areas equally and therefore does not smooth skin (though sometimes spot peeling can be helpful on dark undereye areas). As with dermabrasion, there's always a risk of improper healing and blotchy pigmentary changes in dark-skinned people, especially those of Mediterranean descent, Orientals and blacks. Often, too, chemical peeling produces a different texture to skin (usually lighter, more porcelain, with a finer finish), and so the peeled face may not match the neck, where skin is so delicate it can't take a peel. Thus it may be necessary to wear a foundation all the time and, therefore, I wouldn't recommend it for outdoor, no-makeup, athletic types. (Pregnant women and those with kidney problems are not good candidates either.)

LIGHT ACID CHEMICAL PEELING

Though basically the same procedure as the chemical peel, these peels use a much weaker (and therefore much less potentially risky) acid that is both controllable and highly recommended.

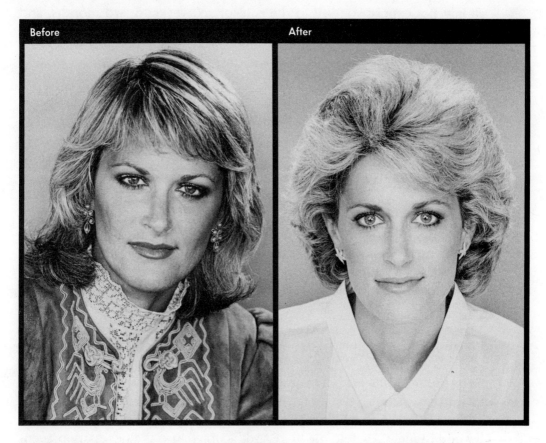

A perfect example of how combining two nonsurgical procedures—a light chemical peel and collagen injections—can take years off your looks. Dr. Allyn Landau did both procedures . . . on herself.

How It Works

Basically this works like the chemical peel. But after the solution is applied, the patient will feel a warm, somewhat tingling sensation, almost like a mild sunburn. The whole procedure takes about twenty minutes.

Recuperation Time

The healing period is approximately three to five days, at which time the superficial layers of the skin are sloughed off (during washing), very much like the peeling that occurs after exposure to the first summer's sun. You should not expose yourself to the sun for six weeks to two months, and when you do, wear a sun screen.

Results

I highly recommend this procedure for reducing pore size, stimulating the growth of new skin cells so skin looks smoother, fresher, younger and for fine crosshatching in weatherbeaten skin (it does not eliminate deep wrinkles). There is no risk of a change in skin tone or texture. The results last for four to six months.

Recommendations/Risks

Even though this is such a fast, simple, dependable and effective procedure, understand that it does take several days for your skin to look presentable enough to appear in public. You can use makeup for camouflage.

ACUPUNCTURE

The acupuncture lift is becoming more and more common. In fact, a California acupuncturist, Dr. Zion Yu (a Chinese-born authority and really the pioneer of the antiwrinkle treatment in this country), regularly treats Hollywood beauties. He told me he regards acupuncture as a necessary preventive procedure that can benefit anyone over thirty.

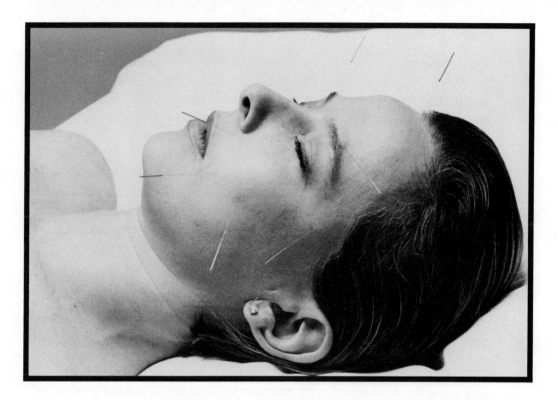

I have to admit I was extremely skeptical about acupuncture as a viable method for getting rid of wrinkles. Nevertheless I tried it (I went to Dr. Yuet Sheung Soong in New York City) and I do believe it can smooth and plump the skin as well as relax facial muscles. (But I have to admit I was so uptight about having needles in my face—and they weren't as painless as they were cracked up to be; some stung!—I left the first treatment more tense than when I arrived. However, I decided to give it another chance, and in the second go-round I was less anxious and could see its potential.) Beyond this, Dr. Soong claims it stimulates circulation, boosts collagen production, causes muscle contractions (and tautness) and brings back a youthful sparkle in the eye—so it could indeed be a useful tool for lessening lines. (I have one friend here in New York City who swears her weekly "lifts" are responsible for her wrinkle-free skin.)

How It Works

The acupuncture lift involves up to thirty superfine, supersharp stainless steel needles (so they don't leave puncture marks) that are inserted slightly below the skin surface in specific spots, mostly on the face. The idea is that the needles release built-up tension in the nerves (you have over 1,000 nerve endings in your face), easing the imbalance of positive and negative forces that cause wrinkles.

Each treatment, which includes the "needling" and usually a massage to condition and moisturize skin, takes about forty-five minutes and is recommended two to three times a week for six to seven weeks. The first ten or so treatments will produce better tone and coloring; the second ten or so will zero in on details—lines around the eyes or lips, say, or on the forehead. After two to three months, maintenance treatments two to three times a month are required to treat specific problems. Prolonged results, though, depend on how well you take care of yourself (acupuncture is based on Oriental precepts of holistic medicine), your general health and how old your skin is. In other words, acupuncture itself doesn't do much good without proper diet, regular exercise and adequate sleep.

Recuperation Time

None. There is no risk of infection and/or swelling.

Results

Acupuncture can ease tension and so diminish expression lines, improve skin tone and texture.

Recommendations/Risks

You'll probably be able to find someone to do the treatment wherever you live, but before you settle on an acupuncturist, I'd look for a diploma of some sort or, better yet, ask for references. Beware of any acupuncturist who makes claims of permanently smoothing skin or who promises immediate results of any sort after only one visit—both are virtually impossible. *Note:* People with extremely wrinkled skin don't get very good results with acupuncture.

LASER LIFTS

Laser physiotherapy, the use of cool laser beams (as opposed to the hot lasers surgeons use), once recommended as an adjunct—the second step, if you will—to acupuncture, is now being considered a major antiaging breakthrough, a procedure in its own right. Research has shown that laser therapy can stimulate collagen production, therefore increasing the strength of the skin so it won't wrinkle.

How It Works

The procedure is painless and involves, quite simply, "beaming" the skin with laser light for five to ten minutes for at least twenty sessions.

Recuperation Time

None. There is no risk of infection or swelling.

Results

Almost immediately the treatment produces a healthy, rosy glow. Plus it's said to improve muscle tone and smooth fine lines, thus also producing tauter, younger-looking skin as it builds the collagen supply to prevent further wrinkling. It will not eliminate jowls or turkey necks.

Recommendations/Risks

The procedure is still in the developmental stages. Yet research is so positive I recommend laser therapy for everyone except drinkers and heavy smokers. *Note:* Do not confuse laser lifts with electric facials (coming right up): Lasers are light treatments, not electric treatments.

ELECTRIC THERAPY

Electric therapy utilizes a machine that administers low-frequency electric currents to facial muscles, tightening them as it increases blood flow, promotes cell rejuvenation and antioxidation (thus decreasing free radicals, cross-linking and the destruction of collagen).

How It Works

Depending on the amount of wrinkling and on your life-style, a full treatment can involve twelve to twenty one-hour visits to an aesthetician. The first week involves two to three visits, the second and third weeks, two each; after that, only one a week. Then, as soon as the treatment is complete, you're put on a maintenance program of one treatment every three to six months. Almost everyone sees and feels a real improvement in the skin after three treatments.

A solution is put on your face to create a "contact" between the skin and the electric current. The first ten minutes are a relaxation period. Then, for

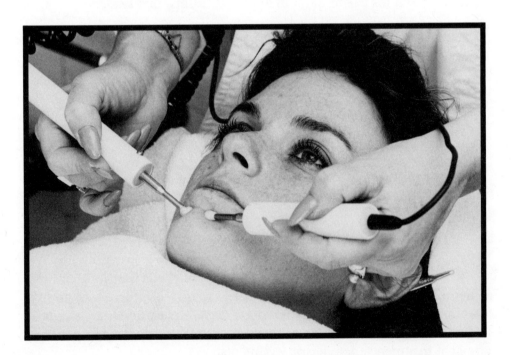

the next forty minutes, two electronic Q-Tiplike probes are rubbed over the face and neck (many patients say the current actually helps them relax, too).

Recuperation Time

None. There's no risk of infection, reddening of skin or swelling. If you experience either, the wrong device or the wrong technique is being used and you should stop treatment immediately.

Results

A quick, easy, no-risk way to restore youthful, healthy skin.

Recommendations/Risks

As with any new and successful technique, there are several knock-off "brands," some of which work and some of which don't. How to tell: The facial machines with high voltages that often burn do not work over the long haul, though they may produce some short-term gains.

CRANIOPATHY OR CRANIAL CONTOURING

It's a unique kind of facial massage, and many famous models and actresses swear by its rejuvenating effects. A manual manipulation of facial muscles firms and recontours droopy faces, sagging cheeks and double chins by toning muscles and realigning facial bones, according to the two practitioners I've consulted. Both are chiropractors (the treatment is an outgrowth of chiropractic medicine). One, Joseph Mirto, is in New York City, and several of my friends have gone to him; the other, Gerald Schneider, is in Beverly Hills and is the choice of lots of celebrities.

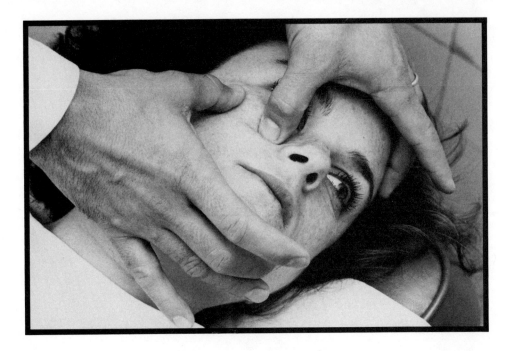

How It Works

Dr. Schneider uses a buffing technique (upward circular strokes) to tone muscles in the face and neck, to increase the blood supply to them and to stimulate the natural moisturizing secretions of the skin—in short, to effect better-looking, younger-looking skin. All it takes: three half-hour weekly visits for three weeks, followed by weekly, then monthly, visits. After ten, you'll see results!

Dr. Schneider has been developing his technique for over fifteen years. It all started in New York City, when a dancer who'd contracted Bell's palsy paralysis in half her face came to him for treatment. In several months the paralyzed side of her face began to look younger than the normal side, and after using his technique on the older-looking "normal" side, it looked as young as the paralyzed side.

Dr. Mirto goes one step further. His technique involves using his hands, both from the inside and outside of the patient's mouth, not only to tone facial muscles weakened by age but to readjust various facial bones that have moved (ever so slightly) because of the weakened muscles and because of organic disturbances caused by, for example, poor nutrition. When the bones are put in their proper positions and the muscles retoned, skin drapes the face more smoothly. Dr. Mirto's treatments don't hurt, take anywhere from five to fifteen minutes and produce noticeable results after six visits.

Recuperation Time

None. There is no risk of infection or swelling.

Results

After several visits you'll see a firmer forehead, tauter cheeks, less of a double chin. Baggy eyes, composed of fatty tissue, not muscle, can't be helped by this treatment.

Recommendations/Risks

Since this is a relatively small branch of chiropractic medicine, there is a relatively small number of practitioners. Make sure yours is for real or you could be wasting your time and money.

Here, to help you get started on your own face, are a few of Dr. Schneider's toners.

1. To smooth forehead frown lines: After bathing, gently rub a damp towel in clockwise circles starting in the center of the forehead, working out, then repeating from the outside in for about a minute.
2. To banish smile lines: Fill cheeks with air and blow out twenty to twenty-five times a day.
3. To erase neck lines: Push chin upward, stretching it as far as you can, and massage neck muscles for five to ten minutes a day.

SEVEN-SECOND EYELID LIFT

It's for real! And it works!

Eyelids are one of the first spots to show aging (they begin to droop and turn crepey), and now, after years of researching a way to solve the problem

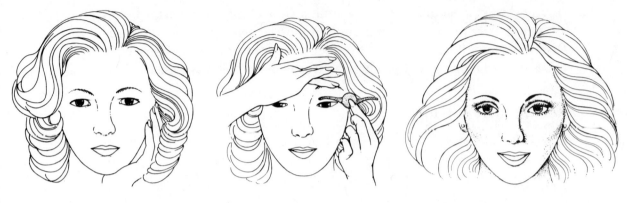

Notice the overhanging eyelids   Applying the double-adhesive tape   Heavy lids disappear instantly

simply and easily, Harold Clavin, M.D., a Santa Monica plastic surgeon, has developed a double-adhesive hypoallergenic upper eyelid tape that lets you effect a temporary blepharosplasty (eye-lift) in a matter of seconds.

How It Works

After removing oil or cosmetics from eyes, you expose the outer adhesive of the correct-size double-face tape, lift it off its liner with its applicator and place it in the desired position on unfolded eyelid skin. (The bottom edge of the tape should be at the desired level of the new fold: Fig. 1.) Then release the tape from the applicator, push the eyebrow down and look up so the skin above the tape folds over it. (Fig. 2.) Pinch eyelid skin together to secure. (Fig. 3.)

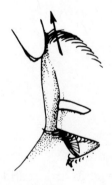

Fig. 1

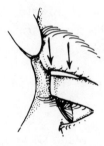

Fig. 2

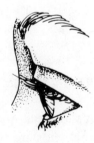

Fig. 3

Recuperation Time

None.

Results

The seven-second eye-lift not only can raise the upper eyelid fold, effecting a younger, wide-eye look, but it can correct asymmetrical upper eyelids, allow for easier, smoother, better makeup application, too.

Recommendations/Risks

It's important to practice with the tape to master the knack of using it (but once you do, it's as easy as applying eyeliner). How high you place the tape determines how high the fold is.

The seven-second lift works wonders on everyone except those with an extremely high eyelid fold, low eyebrows or tight skin.

THE LYMPH MANIPULATION MINILIFT

Widely used in Europe, this treatment is relatively new in the United States, but I can attest to its effectiveness. Soft hand manipulations and vibrations in the lymph node areas on the face, neck and shoulders stimulate internal cleansing (the lymphatic system filters foreign substances and cell debris from the blood and destroys them), relax facial muscles . . . and literally, in a matter of minutes (without creams or machines), smooth facial lines, reduce eye puffiness and fade dark circles. I could hardly believe it!

How It Works

Alla Katov from the Clive Summers Salon in New York City had been calling me for weeks, asking me to try her thirty-minute treatment. I just never had the time. Finally she called one week when my husband and son were off skiing in Colorado and offered to treat me at home after work. I agreed and made arrangements for her to come over one night right before I was going to meet Catherine for dinner.

The treatment was totally relaxing (I fell asleep!) and, I thought, very effective. The proof was Catherine's remark: "It looks like you've found some miracle drug we ought to patent—you look great!"

Recuperation Time

None. There's no risk of swelling or infection.

Results

Smoother, more glowing skin, reduction of undereye puffiness, fading of dark eye circles, calming of sinus discomfort. Results last about a week.

Recommendations/Risks

I'm sold on lymph manipulation. I'd recommend it be incorporated into your life on a weekly basis if you can afford it . . . or at the very least use it "regularly" before a big night or after a particularly stressful day. The only risk: you'll be so relaxed you may want to go right to sleep!

THE "MOUTH LIFT"

If I hadn't talked to Mary F. Riley, D.D.S., a Houston dentist whose practice is devoted largely to cosmetic dentistry, I probably wouldn't have included dentistry as a solution to wrinkles. She convinced me otherwise.

With age, your teeth become shorter, shortening, too, the vertical dimensions of your face and creating lines around lips as well as drooping in the outer corners of the mouth. Dr. Riley told me she builds up front teeth (so they support the lip and "stretch" away lines) with capping and bonding. Bonuses: Capping and bonding also work wonders filling laugh lines, too, and they can make teeth, which become square with age, more oval . . . softer, prettier and more youthful-looking. And Edwin D. Radbill, D.D.S., Catherine's and my dentist here in New York City, says he builds up the back two crowns to lift a droopy mouth.

More dental solutions to aging: As you age, you may notice your gums receding, making your teeth look long, a sign (like short teeth) of your years. Now there's an artificial removable gum insertion that fits over the neck of the tooth, creating the appearance of more gum. It's premade, doesn't require any drilling—it just fits right on! (Bonding can also be used to fill in receding gums.) Tip: The color of your gums should be pink. Massage them daily with the rubber-tipped end of a toothbruth to stimulate circulation; floss regularly, too • Whiter teeth are younger-looking, and today, thanks to greatly advanced bleaching and laminating processes together with capping and bonding, you really have something to smile about. Plus there's a special whitener that comes in two formulas (one with fluoride, one without)—and does it work! You'll see results after one brushing (for smokers it may take up to a week). Developed by Irwin Smigel, D.D.S., president of the American Society for Dental Aesthetics, to remove stains from bonded teeth, it was found to work beautifully on natural teeth, too. It's best used on a dry toothbrush (use water for rinsing only). Ask your dentist if he or she sells it or send for it: Robell Research, 635 Madison Avenue, New York, New York 10022; $8 plus $1.65 shipping and handling for a 4-ounce tube (add local sales tax).

How It Works

Cosmetic dentistry—all the previous processes—can be done in a dentist's office in a matter of hours. Capping requires drilling the tooth down and fitting it with a new, improved, more natural-looking cap or crown (all porcelain rather than the old metal-and-porcelain ones); bonding requires no drilling—simply molding the tooth with a ceramic resin compound; laminating involves covering the tooth with a porcelain veneer; bleaching utilizes a special agent to remove stains. None of this requires Novocain except for capping; and all except capping, which requires several visits, can be done in a single session.

Recuperation Time

None.

Results

A super solution for laugh lines, for diminishing laugh lines, for righting a droopy mouth and for smoothing lines around the lips.

Recommendations/Risks

Make sure your dentist has experience in cosmetic dentistry (ask for references, before-and-after pictures)—you don't want to end up with lopsided caps; bonded, laminated or bleached teeth that mismatch the color of the rest of your teeth; dentures that fit poorly . . . or any one of a number of nonthreatening but definitely irritating results. If you do, don't hesitate to go back for a (free) fix-up, and if that doesn't work, demand a refund and try another dentist. Contact: The American Dental Association, 211 East Chicago Avenue, Chicago, Illinois 60611; (312) 440-2500.

TWO DO-IT-YOURSELF FACE-LIFTS

You just pull away the years!

How They Work

New York City makeup artist Mark Traynor has two ways you can smooth away lines in just a few minutes. One, The Face-Lift, consists of two clear (transparent) adhesive patches and two pieces of elastic. You simply attach the patches to your temples, the elastic to the patches—and then you pull the elastics over your head, join them by hooks, comb your hair over them all . . . and, according to Traynor, take as much as twenty years off your looks.

The second, The Beauty Band Lift: The Beauty Band is an adjustable, 2-inch-wide round of elasticized velour you wear, velour side against your head to keep it firmly in place, like a headband. It's a kind of face girdle.

Recuperation Time

None.

Results

Both lifts smooth the general contours of the face as they smooth fine lines and wrinkles, too. They can be worn as long or as often as you like. The Face-Lift works especially well on laugh lines.

Recommendations/Risks

Mark says you don't have to change your hairstyle to use The Beauty Band, but says it will obviously give you a different look. Plus, you may not be comfortable wearing any kind of hair accessory. (If your hair is very short, you can wear the band with a scarf, turban or wig over it.) To order, write: Mark Traynor, Inc., 114 W. 27th Street, New York, New York 10001. The Beauty Band—$15, The Face-Lift—$8.00, plus $2.50 shipping and handling for both. (New York residents add sales tax.)

FACE INVADERS OF THE BEST KIND

I don't doubt that in considering any of these procedures, you're concerned about how you're going to look afterward (better? worse?). Up until recently all a woman had to go by were photos of other women who'd had the same procedure. But this is all changing.

Dr. Weintraub has helped develop a system (Face Systems, Inc.) that visually shows a patient how he or she will look after an intended procedure. It works this way: A photograph of the patient is taken and the image is transferred onto a computer screen. With an electric pen and a graphics drawing board, Dr. Weintraub can eliminate lines and wrinkles and de-age the face. This means a patient can actually see what she would look like if she were to have a procedure—say, collagen, dermabrasion or a chemical peel—that would make her look years younger.

Two other plastic surgeons, Donald Sklansky, M.D., and Joseph Feinberg, M.D., from Manhasset, Long Island, and New York City, are using videotapes to analyze facial expressions and features to better pinpoint the proper procedure for a patient. For example, a patient might think she needs her nose fixed when, in fact, it's a receding chin that makes her nose look out of whack; or she may come in not knowing what she wants, just knowing she isn't happy with what she looks like now. "Most women don't look at themselves realistically or objectively," Dr. Feinberg told me, "and these videotapes can help them pinpoint what it is they don't like so we can do something about the problem. Plus the tapes can help them eliminate bad facial habits—say, squinting or frowning—they might never have been aware of."

This procedure, too, is used for surgical candidates, but the doctors are looking forward to working with a cosmetologist and a hairstylist to help any patient see how she really looks. Of course, if you have a video machine and camera of your own, you can enlist a friend to help you make your own film.

ANTIAGING MEDICATIONS

Now that you know your physical options for nonsurgical face-lifts, you should consider, too, medicinal options, which are effective on their own or in combination with some of the "lifts" I've just described.

Retin-A

I've tried it—and I like it. Not only did Retin-A actually seem to smooth existing lines over a period of several months, I feel that it's kept my skin looking young and given my complexion a healthy glow. (I've gotten lots of compliments on my skin since I started using it.)

Derived from vitamin A acid, Retin-A, which is primarily used to treat acne, also accelerates cell production, increasing both the number and size of new, healthy skin cells on the stratum corneum and effecting younger-looking, smoother skin. Available by prescription in gel (the mildest concentration), cream and liquid (the most potent) forms, Retin-A is usually applied topically. I recommend you use it under a dermatologist's supervision—he or she can give you a prescription, provide instructions for using it (it can be tricky) on a permanent, preventive basis—and he or she can follow your progress.

The first week I used Retin-A every other day. My skin felt dry and taut, but my doctor told me that was normal. If skin reddens, the Retin-A should be used only every three days the first week, even diluted with equal amounts of a rich moisturizer. (Jonathan Zizmor, M.D., a New York City dermatologist, has a chemist mix the gel form of Retin-A with a moisturizer in a formula weak enough for his patients to use twice a day, A.M. or P.M.) If sensitivity persists, treatment should be stopped altogether.

The second week my skin still felt dry, but I began using the Retin-A once daily at night and I still do. (After week two my skin was back to feeling completely normal.) I usually apply it half an hour before bed (so it won't rub off on the pillow and into my eyes).

Two more tips: If you're traveling from a cold climate to a warm one, stop using Retin-A one week before you go, and once you get there use an SPF of 15 or higher no matter what your skin type. The cold climate you're used to plus the climatic change make skin super sensitive, and the addition of Retin-A makes it sun sensitive, too (see sun-sensitivity section, p. 157). This does not mean you can't use Retin-A in summer; you can. Just apply it at night and rinse your face first thing in the morning before you go outdoors. If you notice any blotching, discontinue use when you're spending time in the sun.

Efudex

Though I don't recommend Efudex, an FDA-approved topical cream or liquid, I think you should be aware of it. It can be a fountain of youth, restoring healthy, youthful skin. Efudex works by destroying old-looking, atypical cells. There is no change in your skin for two weeks, but in the third week your skin will redden; then it will itch, hurt, ulcerate and ooze. The drug is unpredictable (it should never be used by pregnant women or by those who will be exposed to the sun).

Procaine

A local anesthetic (actually a form of Novocain), procaine delivers PABA (para-aminobenzoic acid) to the cells and so protects the skin from cross-linking, particularly that precipitated by exposure to the sun. It's being used by Keith Kenyon, M.D., in Van Nuys, California, to speed cellular metabolism and reduce wrinkles (by tightening support fibers, it flattens superficial lines). It can be administered as an injection or applied topically as a cream. So far it's been simple, safe and extremely effective almost immediately after application. To date it is not sold over the counter.

AND HERE'S WHAT'S AHEAD . . .

- A pill that will convince skin cells they're in their twenties, so they'll behave younger and look younger, too. Research at the National Institute of Health has shown that by removing the pituitary gland of animals, you can make their skin and fur look like that of juveniles.

The hope is to develop a pill that will counter aging controlled by the gland.

· Isolation of certain new amino acids (currently scientists have only isolated 20 percent of those in the body) that have the moisturizing capability of binding water to the skin, as well as skin-toning and firming capabilities.

· Identification of the agent—the "Tissue Control Factor" currently under investigation at the University Genetics Company in Norwalk, Connecticut—that controls the rate at which cells replace themselves. The good news: Scientists have been able to stop aging altogether in lab cells.

· The development of androgen blockers—synthetic compounds that will increase production of skin-firming elastin.

· New advances and applications for artificial skin now being used to treat burn victims.

TEN

THE WRINKLE FIXERS:
WHERE TO GO
FOR WHAT

Because I'm so frequently asked to recommend doctors and beauty experts, I decided to compile a list of those used in this book. Here they are, chapter by chapter, complete with addresses and telephone numbers.

Chapter 1

Susan M. Lark, M.D.
PMS Self Help Center
170 State Street
Los Altos, CA 94022
(415) 941-1540

Schick Center For Control of Smoking
20 centers
(213) 553-3366

Chapter 2

James R. White, Ph.D.
Department of Physical Education
University of California at San Diego
La Jolla, CA 92093
(619) 452-4030

Chapter 3

Albert M. Kligman, M.D., Ph.D.
Department of Dermatology
University of Pennsylvania School
of Medicine
244 Medical Education Building
36th and Hamilton Walk
Philadelphia, PA 19104
(215) 898-3230

Darrell Rigel, M.D.
213 Madison Avenue
New York, NY 10016
(212) 684-5964

Chapter 4

Ian S. Brown, M.D.
465 North Roxbury Drive
Beverly Hills, CA 90210
(213) 858-1505

Ruth Domber
10/10 Optics
1010 Second Avenue
New York, NY 10022
(212) 753-7733

Frank S. Socha, M.D.
240 East 64th Street
New York, NY 10021
(212) 308-1566

Chapter 5

Mister Lee Hair Stylist
834 Jones Street
San Francisco, CA 94109
(415) 474-6002

Charles Nicholas Hair Salon
48 East 57th Street
New York, NY 10022
(212) 355-1133

Chapter 6

Meredith L. Hoblock, M.S., R.D.
90 Prince Street
New York, NY 10012
(212) 807-4140

Hermien Lee, M.S.
9401 Wilshire Boulevard
Beverly Hills, CA 90212
(213) 276-7491

Carl C. Pfeiffer, M.D., Ph.D.
Princeton Brain Bio Center
862 Route 518
Skillman, NJ 08558
(609) 924-8607

Sonoma Mission Inn and Spa
18140 Sonoma Highway 12
Boyes Hot Springs, CA 95416
(707) 938-9000

Chapter 8

Adriana's Skin Care
34 East 67th Street
New York, NY 10021
(212) 772-0488

Christiana and Carmen Skin Care
Salon
128 Central Park South
New York, NY 10019
(212) 757-5811

T. J. D'Ifray Institut de Beauté
468 North Bedford Drive
Beverly Hills, CA 90210
(213) 274-6776

Aida Grey Institut de Beauté
9549 Wilshire Boulevard
Beverly Hills, CA 90212
(213) 276-2376

The Beverly Wilshire Hotel
9500 Wilshire Boulevard
Beverly Hills, CA 90212
(213) 550-9827

Ole Henriksen of Denmark Skin Care
Center
8601 West Sunset Boulevard
Los Angeles, CA 90069
(213) 854-7700

Hippocrates Health Institute
25 Exeter Street
Boston, MA 02116
(617) 267-9525

Ilona of Hungary Institutes of Skin
Care
629 Park Avenue
New York, NY 10021
(212) 288-5155

3201 East Second Avenue
Denver, CO 80206
(303) 322-4212

45 East Oak Street
Chicago, IL 60611
(312) 337-7161

1800 South Post Oak Boulevard
Houston, TX 77056
(713) 961-4844

Kerstin Skin Care
1465 South Coast Highway
Laguna Beach, CA 92651
(714) 497-4868

Georgette Klinger Skincare Salons
501 Madison Avenue
New York, NY 10022
(212) 838-3200

978 Madison Avenue
New York, NY 10021
(212) 744-6900

312 North Rodeo Drive
Beverly Hills, CA 90210
(213) 274-6347

The Galleria
13350 Dallas Parkway
Dallas, TX 75240
(214) 385-9393

Water Tower Place
835 North Michigan Avenue
Chicago, IL 60611
(312) 787-4300

Bal Harbour Shops
9700 Collins Avenue
Bal Harbour, FL 33154
(305) 868-7516

Esplanade
150 Worth Avenue
Palm Beach, FL 33480
(305) 659-1522

Klisar Skin Care Center
18 East 53rd Street
New York, NY 10022
(212) 838-4422

Christine Kunzelman
Panache Appearance Studios
3902 Pacific Coast Highway
Torrance, CA 90505
(213) 378-8308

Ingrid Millet Institut de Beauté
54, rue du Faubourg Saint-Honoré
75008 Paris, France
011-33-1-266-66-20

Ingrid Millet Institut de Beauté at
Henri Bendel
10 West 57th Street
New York, NY 10019
(212) 247-1100

Laura Norman & Associates
2 East 37th Street
New York, NY 10016
(212) 532-4404

Lia Schorr Skin Care
686 Lexington Avenue
New York, NY 10022
(212) 486-9670

Peter Stephan's Center
27 Harley Place
Harley Street, London W1
01-636-6197

Livia Sylva Bee Pollen Clinic de Beauté
133 East 54th Street
New York, NY 10022
(212) 759-9797

Aida Thibiant Skin and Body Care
Center
449 North Canon Drive
Beverly Hills, CA 90210
(213) 278-7565

Christine Valmy's Skin Care Salons
G M Plaza
767 Fifth Avenue
New York, NY 10153
(212) 752-0303

153 West 57th Street
New York, NY 10019
(212) 581-9488

1 Rockefeller Plaza
Concourse Level
New York, NY 10020
(212) 315-4141

107-27 71st Avenue
Forest Hills, NY 11375
(718) 793-0222

Diane Young Skin Care Center
243 East 60th Street
New York, NY 10022
(212) 753-1200

The Super Spas

Ashram Health Resort
Box 8009
Calabasas, CA 91302
(818) 888-0232

Canyon Ranch Spa
8600 East Rockcliff Road
Tucson, AZ 85715
(602) 749-9000

Clinic La Prairie
CH-1815 Clarens-Montreux
Switzerland
(212) 772-8470

Filion's Health and Beauty Spa
King Edward Hotel
37 King Street East
Toronto, Ontario, Canada M5C1E9
(416) 365-1433

Gerovital Treatment Tours
Romanian National Tourist Office
573 Third Avenue
New York, NY 10016
(212) 697-6971

The Golden Door
Box 1567
Escondido, CA 92025
(619) 744-5777

Maine Chance
5830 East Jean Avenue
Phoenix, AZ 85018
(602) 947-6365

Quiberon Institute
Pointe de Gouvars
56170 Quiberon, France
(97) 50-20-00

Rancho La Puerta
Tecate, Baja California
Mexico KM5
Ranch: (706) 654-1155
Reservations: (619) 478-5341

Spa at the Hotel Plantation de Leyritz
97218 Basse-Pointe, Martinique
FWI
(596) 75-5392

Terme di Montecatini
Viale Verdi, 41
51016 Montecatini Terme, Italy
011-39-572-75801

Chapter 9

Acupuncture

Dr. Yuet Sheung Soong
1035 Park Avenue
New York, NY 10028
(212) 369-5263

Dr. Zion Yu
Kinetic Medical Center
16055 Ventura Boulevard
Encino, CA 91436
(818) 905-5506

Antiaging medications

Jonathan Zizmor, M.D.
655 Park Avenue
New York, NY 10021
(212) 688-8326

Collagen

Craig Foster, M.D.
1016 Fifth Avenue
New York, NY 10028
(212) 744-5746

Allyn Landau, M.D.
260 Stockton Street
San Francisco, CA 94108
(415) 781-2122

Craniopathy or cranial contouring

Joseph Mirto, D.C.
580 Park Avenue
New York, NY 10021
(212) 838-6600

Gerald Schneider
8530 Wilshire Boulevard
Beverly Hills, CA 90211
(213) 657-7523

Electric Therapy

Elyse Grant
Institute of Body Esthetics
P.O. Box 64
Glastonbury, CT 06033
(203) 649-0080

Face Invaders of the Best Kind

Donald Sklansky, M.D.
Joseph Feinberg, M.D.
1201 Northern Boulevard
Manhasset, NY 11030
(516) 869-8282

475 East 72nd Street
New York, NY 10021
(212) 744-9080

Barry Weintraub, M.D.
145 South Rodeo Drive
Beverly Hills, CA 90212
(213) 278-7277

Fibrel

Gary D. Monheit, M.D.
1717 11th Avenue South
Birmingham, AL 35205
(205) 933-0987

The Lymph Manipulation Minilift

Alla Katov
Clive Summers Salon
645 Fifth Avenue
New York, NY 10022
(212) 751-7501

The Mouth Lift

Edwin D. Radbill, D.D.S.
654 Madison Avenue
New York, NY 10021
(212) 838-8363

Mary F. Riley, D.D.S.
5 Post Oak Park
Houston, TX 77027
(713) 622-1707

The Muscle Relaxing Injectable Forehead Lift

Stephen Genender, M.D.
8635 West 3rd Street
Los Angeles, CA 90048
(213) 659-5502

Procaine

Dr. Keith Kenyon
Beverly Hills Rejuvenation Medical
Center
Electro Nutrition Clinic
14435 Hamlin Street
Van Nuys, CA 91401
(818) 782-2820

Seven-second Eyelid Lift

Harold Clavin, M.D.
2001 Santa Monica Boulevard
Santa Monica, CA 90404
(213) 829-5977

Makeovers

Gad Cohen
(212) 517-7604

Craig Gadson
(212) 223-3774

Hair by Garren for Garren, New York
(212) 686-5277

Aldo Giacomello
Kenneth Salon
19 East 54th Street
New York, NY 10022
(212) 752-1800

Francois Ilnseher
(212) 245-0200

Louis Licari
La Coupe Salon
694 Madison Avenue
New York, NY 10021
(212) 371-9230

Sandy Linter
(212) 925-8552

Pablo Manzoni Makeup Consultations
Ritz Tower
465 Park Avenue
New York, NY 10022
(212) 355-5700

Cida Nery
Kenneth Salon
19 East 54th Street
New York, NY 10022
(212) 752-1800